STRETCHING
WITH **EASE**

An illustrated guide to your **fit** and **flexible** body

Linda Minarik

Foreword by Brad Walker
Author of *The Anatomy of Stretching*

CICO BOOKS
LONDON NEW YORK

For Dalmo and Dan, who always believed in me.

And for my Dad, in gratitude for his love and bravery.

Published in 2015 by CICO Books
an imprint of Ryland Peters & Small Ltd
20–21 Jockey's Fields, London WC1R 4BW
341 E 116th St, New York, NY 10029

www.rylandpeters.com

10 9 8 7 6 5 4 3 2 1

Text © Linda Minarik 2015
Foreword © Brad Walker 2015
Design and photography © CICO Books 2015

Please note that the information in this book should not be substituted for advice from your physician. If you have any health concerns, consult your physician for guidance before doing any of the exercises in this book. The publisher and the author cannot be held responsible for any health issue that may arise indirectly or directly from the use of this book.

A CIP catalog record for this book is available from the Library of Congress and the British Library.

ISBN: 978 1 78249 263 4

Printed in China

Editor: Jane Birch
Designer: Isobel Gillan
Photographer and illustrator: Rob Zeller

Commissioning editor: Kristine Pidkameny
In-house editor: Dawn Bates
In-house designer: Fahema Khanam
Art director: Sally Powell
Production controller: David Hearn
Publishing manager: Penny Craig
Publisher: Cindy Richards

Contents

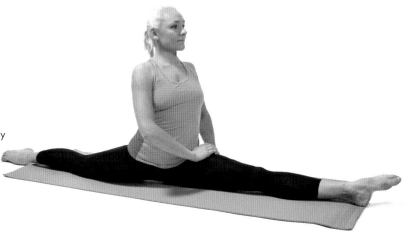

contents

5

contents

Foreword

My interest in stretching and flexibility began in 1987 when I was introduced to the sport of triathlon. Back then, reliable information on the topic of stretching was almost non-existent, so I spent the next five years testing and experimenting on myself and other athletes.

One of my strengths in this field is that I have been fortunate enough to work with many different athletes from many different sports; everything from baseball and squash to motorcycle racing, roller skating, and triathlon, as well as regular, everyday people who just want to improve their mobility and freedom of movement. This gives me a perspective on stretching and flexibility that very few other people have.

And I believe this is one of the strengths that Linda brings to her new publication: *Stretching with Ease*.

Being able to draw on her background in dance and combine that with her experience in karate, aerobics, and yoga—plus her knowledge of the Gyrokinesis® method, The MELT® Method, and the Alexander Technique—put her in a unique position: a big-picture position.

Many people make the mistake of seeing stretching as a narrow, isolated activity. They put stretching in a box and only open that box when something goes wrong, like an injury, or they have some spare time.

Linda, on the other hand, sees stretching from a holistic, big-picture perspective. She is able to draw on her 20-plus years of experience and weave stretching into all aspects of movement and fitness.

Linda's new publication follows a very common-sense approach, first outlining the "who," "what," "why," "when," and "how" of stretching. It then goes on to give clear examples of different stretches for different muscle groups, sports, and pain points; and finishes by giving you tools to make stretching a regular part of your everyday life.

So read, learn, and enjoy *Stretching with Ease*. But most important, apply it and weave it into your everyday life.

BRAD WALKER
AKA the Stretch Coach
Author of *The Anatomy of Stretching*
and the *Ultimate Guide to Stretching*

Preface

My personal quest for flexibility has now lasted over 20 years. When it began, everyone from dance to karate to gymnastics to mainstream fitness talked about stretching, but there was precious little organized instruction accessible to someone who spent her growing-up years sitting at the piano and was now looking to get flexible. Either you were flexible or you weren't, it seemed, and those who were seemed in possession of some great secret. Even today, talk to a dancer and you will still likely encounter the attitude: "If you weren't flexible growing up, forget it now, honey."

Too often have I been pronounced too old to accomplish X, Y, or Z (fill in your own X), and I did not take this lying down. Slowly—asking questions; practicing stretching with what knowledge I could garner; seeking out people who thought, as I dared to, that a flexible body could be had at any age with the right knowledge and training—I started unraveling the mystery of how one becomes truly flexible. Now, more than 20 years later, I can proudly say I am much more flexible than ever before. I have awareness of and can move my sacrum; standing with my palms flat on the floor is positively easy; and I am well on the way to having a split.

While my own journey continues to unfold, I have been teaching group fitness continuously since 1993—logging thousands of hours helping people get the most from their fitness education. Over the last seven years or so, I have been developing an expertise in teaching the art of flexibility to the non-fitness-professional enthusiasts in my classes. They take time from their stressful day to refresh themselves by working with their bodies. How could I create a worthwhile stretching experience for this fitness audience—giving them the needed basics and yet respecting their intelligence? Gradually I began to formulate an effective teaching language.

The more I taught, the clearer my instructions became, and my classes began to grow in size. I passed on all the hard-won knowledge I had unearthed over more than two decades of searching. This book represents a distillation and compilation of my teaching experience.

Studies exist that examine various aspects of the stretching experience, and I have done some reading along scientific, theoretical lines. But the groundwork for this book is laid using the empirical research approach. I have verified the effects of various stretching techniques through my own observations and experience, as well as those of colleagues I have consulted.

I saw the invitation to write this book as a chance to expose a wider audience to what I have learned and have been privileged to share with others. Putting the right words on the page to convey to a reader the magic of a body and mind working together on their common goal of increasing flexibility has been an enormous challenge. I have done my best to meet it.

It is my hope that the ideas you find in this book will shed some light on your own pursuit of flexibility, and perhaps spark a deep appreciation for the amazing opportunity human beings have to live in the marvelous bodies we possess.

May the stars shine upon the end of your road.

Introduction

What is flexibility?

Defining flexibility is not that simple. I have just looked through four books on stretching that I consulted as references for this text. None of them defines flexibility. *The Shorter Oxford English Dictionary* does not even treat this word in a human-body context. When I mentioned flexibility in my stretching classes, students have asked me, "What's that?"

And yet, flexibility is what we are after when we stretch our muscles. Consider this definition:

Flexibility is the freedom we have to move with as great a range of motion, in all our body parts, as we need for any activity we want to undertake.

In other words:

- **For daily life** you need enough flexibility to bend down and pick up something you dropped on the floor.
- **For aerobic dance** you need enough flexibility to lift your knee to 90 degrees without tucking your pelvis under.
- **For gymnastics** you need enough flexibility to execute a split.

Whatever you want to accomplish—however simple or complex the movement—possessing adequate flexibility means you can do it easily, without a struggle. Stretching is what you do to acquire that flexibility.

The pursuit of flexibility is a vast, bottomless-pit topic. One book cannot hope to cover all the ins and outs, permutations, and prestidigitations of this field of study. An entire book could be written on any of the subjects briefly discussed in this one. There is so much to say about flexibility and its benefits that trying to do it some kind of justice in the space here allotted is a hugely daunting task.

What you will find here, though, is a jumping-off place for your personal research. You will get enough information to provide you with a mental foothold as you begin to explore using flexibility to bring some benefit into your life—but not enough information to overwhelm you. You do not need any previous experience with stretching to employ the knowledge presented here. If you are already an experienced stretching practitioner, the clear instructions offered can help you organize the knowledge you have, and maybe give you some ideas for next steps in your quest for ever-greater freedom of movement.

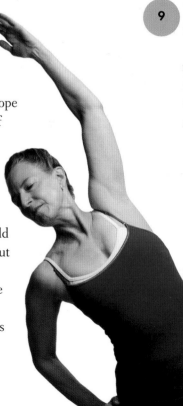

Some things to consider as you begin

- **Flexibility is specific.** If you can bend over and put your palms on the ground, that's great, but it doesn't guarantee that you can open your knees wide to the side in a kneeling position. You may have a fairly good range of motion when you do a stretch on one side of your body, and a curtailed range when you try it on the other.

  Specificity means that, to gain body-wide flexibility—and hence ease of motion—you must stretch each area separately. Flexibility doesn't automatically transfer to the opposite side or to other body parts. Unfortunately, there are no shortcuts in flexibility training. (Don't panic—it's not all work and no play. Practicing stretching will make you feel *really* good.)

- **Flexibility is one component of a comprehensive physical fitness regimen.** A flexible body—of paramount importance for health and athletics—is still only one of a number of aspects of your complete fitness program. Brad Walker gives a good catalogue of these:

  Other components include strength, power, speed, endurance, balance, coordination, agility, and skill.[1]

If you are a non-professional fitness participant, you will probably place less importance on power, speed, agility, and skill. But for health (and to negotiate in the world), everyone needs some degree of strength, endurance, coordination, and balance. For example, weight training addresses strength; cardiovascular training endurance. Your flexibility practice will work in concert with the other prongs of your fitness program.

Conventions used in this book

Part Two: Your Stretch Repertory

- **Sports injury list.** At the beginning of each chapter in this section is a selection of sports injuries that the stretches discussed might help to heal. The list is not comprehensive; neither are the injuries defined. They are terms in common use, and will be familiar to many readers. The injuries mentioned will be most relevant if you have been "diagnosed" with one of these conditions as a result of pain in an area: you will recognize the name and be able to use the appropriate stretches.

- **Stretch descriptions.** We describe each of the 73 stretches referenced in this section for one side of your body only. All tips and thoughts are oriented to this first side. When you stretch the other side, just switch the words "right" and "left."

Part Three: Stretch Sequences—Stretch Before and After Common Physical Activities

Stretching can enhance any physical activity, but we limit this discussion to a selection of activities that a non-professional participant might be likely to engage in as exercise. Photographs show stretches helpful for playing basketball, because basketball is one of the sports covered in this section. But you can adapt these stretches for other ball sports as well, for example, volleyball. Similarly with the discussion of racquetball/handball: the stretches mentioned are useful for tennis and other racquet sports as well. (Tennis gets its own little addendum within the section.) In general, the muscles used for swinging the racquet are similar to those used in throwing. And golf, the king of torso-rotation sports, is referenced, though not extensively discussed.

In conclusion

Your experience is your own—and only your own. Never discount its validity. No one can know what will benefit you better than you do. Ask advice of others; consult books like this one. When all the evidence is in, the best decisions about how to proceed are rightfully yours. You are the person best qualified to give yourself an optimal stretching experience, because only you can cultivate an open exchange of feelings and ideas between your marvelous body and mind.

The more time, effort, and study you devote to stretching, the greater chance you have of realizing your body's maximum flexibility potential—which is quite a lot. Seeking a high degree of skill in this art is the work of a lifetime. Realize that your chronological "age" is not relevant (see *Part One: What Muscles to Stretch*, p. 36, and *Part Four: Supporting Flexibility*, p. 178). What your body cares about is your *biological age*—your degree of health. If you are not limber now, you can become so—with the right combination of elements. You need belief, passion, and unrelenting action—with these, nothing can stop you.

Consider this quote, still applicable today, from one of the best films ever made:

I believe in the pursuit of excellence, and I'll carry the future with me.
—*Chariots of Fire*

That's what this book is about, and that's what I wish for your life.

Start now. Jump in. A whole new world awaits when you turn the page.

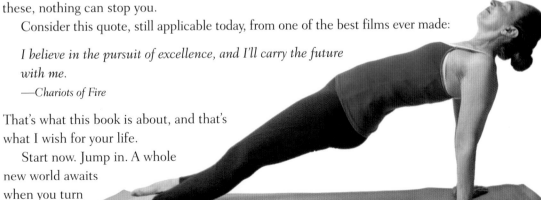

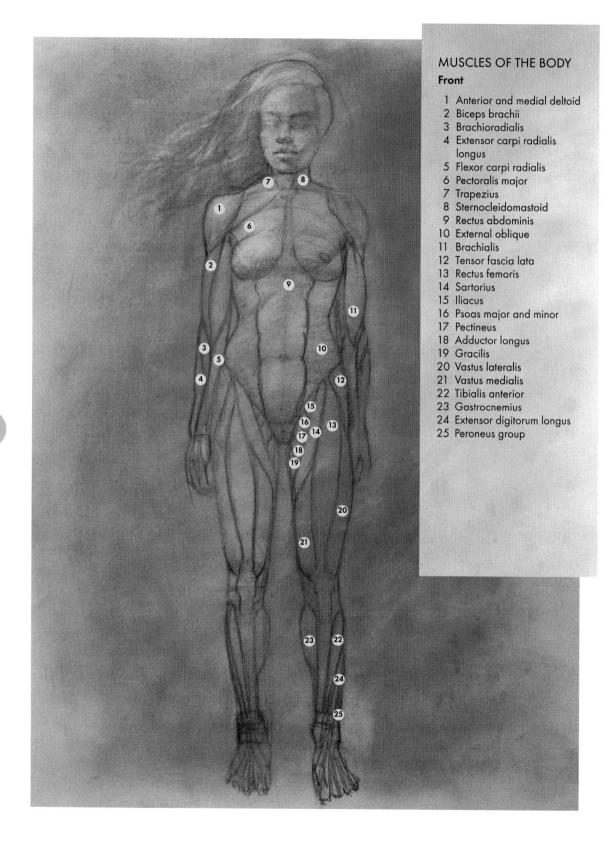

MUSCLES OF THE BODY
Front

1 Anterior and medial deltoid
2 Biceps brachii
3 Brachioradialis
4 Extensor carpi radialis longus
5 Flexor carpi radialis
6 Pectoralis major
7 Trapezius
8 Sternocleidomastoid
9 Rectus abdominis
10 External oblique
11 Brachialis
12 Tensor fascia lata
13 Rectus femoris
14 Sartorius
15 Iliacus
16 Psoas major and minor
17 Pectineus
18 Adductor longus
19 Gracilis
20 Vastus lateralis
21 Vastus medialis
22 Tibialis anterior
23 Gastrocnemius
24 Extensor digitorum longus
25 Peroneus group

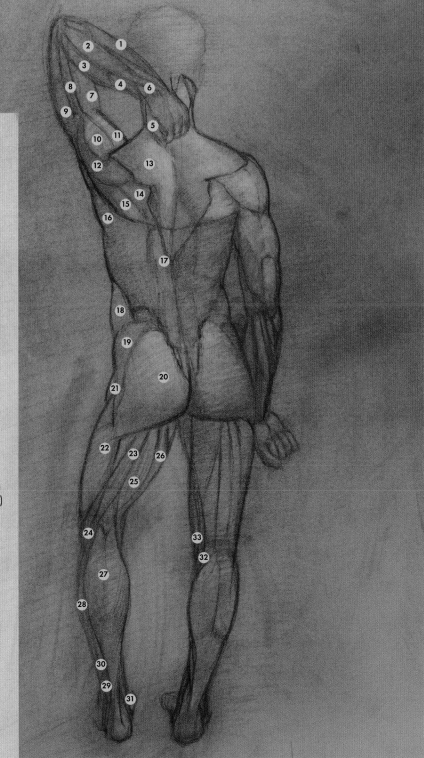

MUSCLES OF THE BODY
Back

1 Extensor carpi ulnaris
2 Extensor digitorum
3 Extensor carpi radialis
   longus
4 Abductor pollicis longus
5 Abductor pollicis brevis
6 Extensor pollicis longus
7 Biceps brachii
8 Brachialis
9 Triceps
10 Medial deltoid
11 Anterior deltoid
12 Posterior deltoid
13 Trapezius
14 Infraspinatus
15 Teres major
16 Latissimus dorsi
17 Erector spinae
18 External oblique
19 Gluteus medius
20 Gluteus maximus
21 Tensor fascia lata
22 Vastus lateralis
23 Biceps femoris (long head)
24 Biceps femoris (short head)
25 Semitendinosus
26 Semimembranosus
27 Gastrocnemius
28 Soleus
29 Flexor hallucis longus
30 Peroneus group
31 Flexor digitorum longus
32 Gracilis
33 Sartorius

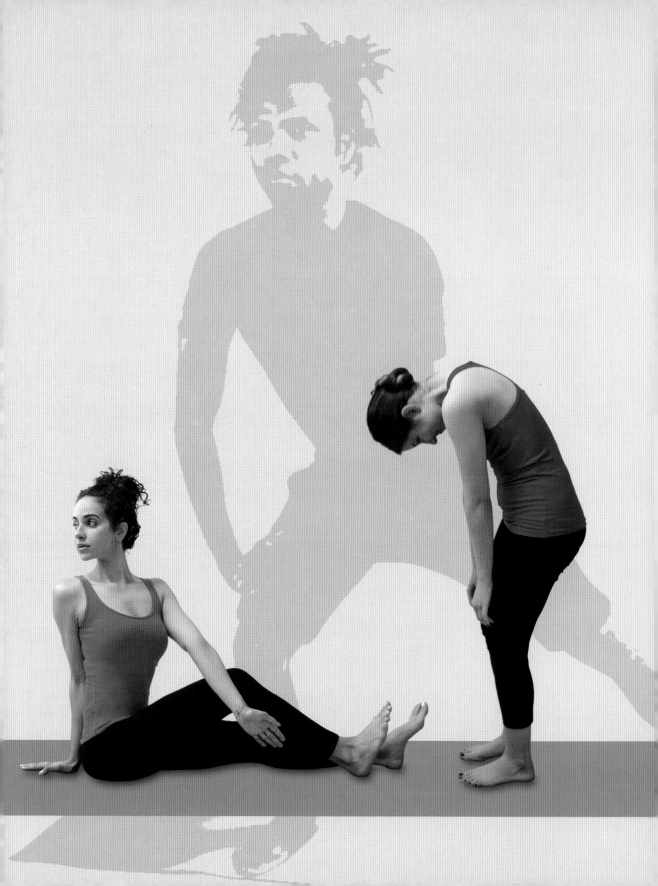

PART ONE
BEFORE YOU STRETCH

You are the master of the partnership between your body and your mind. Like many people who take my flexibility classes, you are pursuing excellent personal fitness. Perhaps you are not a professional in fitness, but you are certainly a professional elsewhere in your life. You have job experience that is irreplaceable, or a combination of personal and workplace qualities shared by no one else. Acknowledge your unique qualities, and bring them to flexibility training. This group of articles will introduce you to some solid logic behind the study of stretching. Get your discerning mind behind learning how to stretch correctly and well, and you will increase your chances of successfully—and permanently—incorporating a beneficial flexibility practice into your life. I hope that the material in this section will afford you the right impetus to launch that practice.

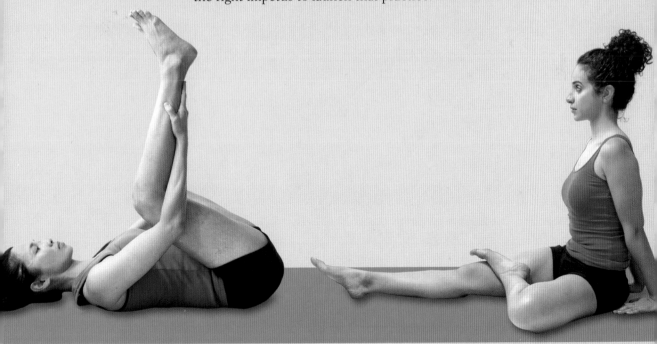

Why stretch?

Why would you take time from an incredibly busy life for a slow activity like stretching? Life is full of demands on every side. Many professional people start work early and get home late. Busy moms find their days broken up by driving kids to multiple activities. Time is at a premium—for everyone. Entertain the possibility that inserting a stretch and a breath into an odd free moment can make all the hustle seem less hectic.

Our days of hunting and gathering, and spending our days tracking, killing, and cooking food—or else outrunning the proverbial saber-tooth tiger—may be behind us, but the myth that modern conveniences make our fast-paced, worldwide-web lives simpler is just that: a myth.

We no longer have to fear becoming a tiger's dinner, but there are still plenty of tiger stand-ins around to trigger our fight-or-flight responses. And our systems are hard-wired: they react the same way to a high-pressure work deadline as they would to a prehistoric tiger.

The techniques you will learn in this book have the capacity to take you farther along the road to true relaxation than you would get by merely stretching a muscle or only quieting the mind. By joining thought, body awareness, and movement, it is possible to create a space inside yourself where the pressures bearing on you do not exist. Even if you can spare only ten minutes, choosing techniques from those offered that benefit your unique makeup most can be enough to dissipate the negative effects of stress, help to prevent injury, relieve pain and muscular soreness, improve your posture and level of well-being, and up your athletic ability. Life will still be there when you emerge from your stretching space, but you will be much better equipped to face it.

I invite you to create an interior magic bubble where life's overriding concerns do not reach you. Although you cannot recover or replace the resource of time, I invite you to devote a little of the time you have to something that has the potential to make the rest of it calmer, better-feeling, and more efficient—stretching.

Benefit 1: stretching reduces and heals stress

Stress is a very real "aging" agent. Negative stress in its many incarnations is alive and well and with us in the 21st century—as the briefest glance at your life will show. And one thing you can do to counteract its evil effects is—stretch.

For the body to increase its range of muscle movement, it must calm down. Your body is very often in "alert" mode, constantly looking over its shoulder, so to speak, to make sure it is safe. Such a never-ending state of stress does not advance optimum health. But how can you dissipate this state? Just see what happens

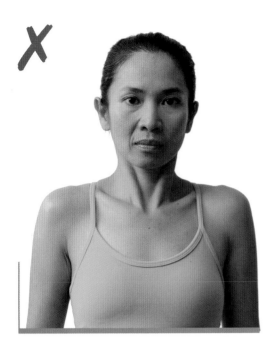

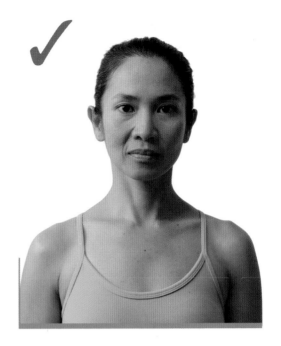

when you put your body into a flexibility class, lie down on the floor, and use the exhale phase of your breath to allow a particular muscle to relax and lengthen. When you exhale, your body gets the message, "It is safe to relax. I am in a safe place." Your body can start to open up and increase its muscular range—but not if it isn't convinced it has nothing to fear. By definition, when the body is able to increase muscle range of movement, your nervous system uses the parasympathetic—relaxing—branch of the autonomic nervous system (ANS). You are less likely to trigger the go-on-alert branch of the ANS—the sympathetic. You experience fewer detrimental effects from stress. Your stress level goes down.

Benefit 2: stretching prevents injury

Injury prevention—a pair of words you might struggle to get your mind around. These words have been used so often they may border on useless jargon. Here's a simple situation you can envision.

At some time in your life you may have done something called "turning your ankle." Accidentally, of course. It takes you unawares. Suddenly you're on the floor in pain, and you end up with a swollen ankle. In my high school basketball days, I was so familiar with this situation that I actually started wearing ACE™ bandages over my ankles to every practice.

The ankle always turns on the outside of your foot—never the inside. Try this. Stand with your feet side by side and let your right ankle drop outside—to the right. It goes over rather easily. Now drop it inside—to the left. It doesn't go there, right? The ankle has much more tendency to collapse out than in. That's your vulnerable spot.

Now, let's say you did the following stretch twice a week for two months.

Sit down in a chair and place your right ankle on your left thigh. Let your right knee open. Now, gently stretch the right ankle into the "turned-ankle" position and hold for 30 seconds. Experience the stretchy feeling, but stop short of actual pain. No forcing. Repeat three times. Then repeat on the other ankle. Your investment of time for this is about five minutes. You can do it while you are (famously) watching TV.

The next time you turn your ankle (always a shock), your ankle will be capable of displacing itself farther from its home position without harm. The stretch has prevented an injury.

The same principle applies to other stretches as well. Think of the golfer's swing and how his spine must twist—both in the wind-up and the release. If he rotates his spine on a regular basis, his body will not feel it is doing anything out of the ordinary, and therefore won't injure itself during the move. The philosophy is: don't wait until an injury occurs. Add this new dimension to your fitness program now.

Benefit 3: stretching relieves pain

One important place to experience this effect is in the area of low-back pain, often exacerbated by tight hamstrings (muscles in the back of your thighs). The low back and sacrum (spine below your waist) cause many people pain. Although many doctors are of the opinion that the sacral vertebrae are "fused" and operate totally as a unit, the fact is that there is a little movement available in that area. If people learn techniques to increase that movement ability gently, freeing the vertebrae from constriction while they also loosen up the hamstring muscles, the pain can be reduced or eliminated.

The connection of tight hamstrings with back pain is a good case in point, because tight hamstrings stop the hips from flexing during forward bending, forcing the lower back to bend beyond its strong middle range. This is the sort of

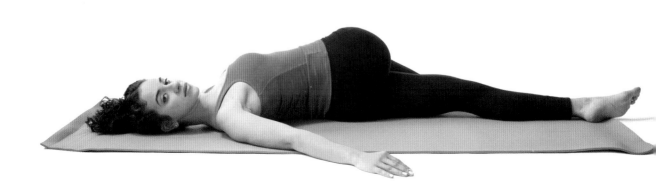

thing that may happen in a yoga class, if the teacher is not knowledgeable enough to spot and correct it. The back over-stretches to accommodate tight hamstrings, and the problem (and the pain) may just get worse. If you work in an office, the constant chair-sitting you do is already contributing to this problem, even before you add any exercises that work hamstrings—which makes them tighter.

The same principle applies to improving mobility in other areas. Hence, a stretching program can go far toward relieving pain. It can also happen that one part of the body becomes tight, and another part compensates: you feel the tightness in the compensating area. When you stretch one area—such as the upper back—pain may be relieved in another area—such as the lower back.

Benefit 4: stretching relieves muscular soreness

You are probably familiar with what is termed "post-exercise muscle soreness." When you work muscles you are not used to using, or work your muscles at a different angle, they get sore a day or two days later. There are dietary measures and supplements you can take to reduce this soreness, but when you do experience it, stretching can come to the rescue.

After reading this book, you will be familiar with what muscles are located where in your body, what it feels like to stretch each particular muscle group, and what stretches to do when you are confronted with muscle soreness in an area. In this respect, you can become your own physical therapist or personal trainer. You will have knowledge that allows you to remedy the little soreness glitches your body may develop as you go along living your life and doing your fitness program of choice.

Benefit 5: stretching improves posture and body symmetry

Your ability to move your body easily in any direction you wish can be impaired by habitual actions, like:

- Emphasis on working only one side of the body—such as arm wrestling. One arm becomes much stronger than the other.

- Emphasis on working one muscle group to the exclusion of another. When bodybuilders emphasize the bench press (chest) more than back exercises, the chest muscles become strong and tight and can round the shoulders forward.

- Sitting with shoulders rounded forward—again shortening the chest muscles and weakening the back muscles that should work to keep the shoulders centered.

Working and stretching both sides of the body provide a good solution for situations like these.

Benefit 6: stretching advances physical and athletic skills

Whatever your area of athletic endeavor, a high degree of flexibility is in your favor. Take a look at the possibilities:

- It's absolutely necessary for skilled, artistic movement ability, as in dance, gymnastics, or karate. Michael Alter says it best:

  Flexibility allows the individual to create an appearance of ease, smoothness of movement, graceful coordination, self-control, and total freedom.... Flexibility can provide the critical difference between average and outstanding performance.[1]

  Who wouldn't want that?

- A greater range of motion will give an athlete's movement more force, speed, momentum. A baseball pitcher can reach farther back when he winds up to throw if his shoulder's rotator-cuff muscles are flexible. (A flexible core doesn't hurt either.) In the weight-training context, the best-stretched muscle is capable of the hardest work.

Of course, the converse is: not enough flexibility can impair athletic movement. If an athlete's hips are not flexible enough to permit free movement, she can have lower-back issues. She can reverse this by gaining greater freedom in her hips using stretching.

The bottom line is:

Quality of movement is either enhanced by flexibility or constrained by the lack of it.[2]

In conclusion: the case for flexibility training

A well-balanced fitness program includes at least the three prongs of resistance, aerobic, and flexibility training. Unfortunately, flexibility seems to be the prong often neglected by the exercise participant. When time is short, it is much easier to feel that you worked out by doing 30 minutes of aerobic training or hitting the machines than by doing 30 minutes of work on lengthening your body's muscles.

In my 20+ years as a group fitness instructor and personal trainer, I have witnessed the heroic efforts gym members make to pursue fitness programs in the face of many challenges. I've seen women devote their lunch hour on a regular basis to a cardiovascular or weight-training class, making sure that fitness is a part of their day. Some have a two-hour commute each way; yet they make fitness a priority. I've seen people show up at the gym at 6 a.m. or 7 a.m., because working out before they report for their jobs is the only time they have. I've seen people come in on weekends, traveling a distance to take a class at an inconvenient time because they care so much about their fitness level. I totally get that hard choices are necessary when you are selecting efficient workouts for a tightly scheduled life.

Still, it remains that balancing hard-core, high-energy workouts with stretching ones is important for a high overall fitness level. When muscles are constantly worked, they shorten and, if not systematically lengthened again through stretching, can remain that way, to such an extent that bones are pulled out of line and poor posture—not to mention pain—results.

In addition to balancing other types of workouts, correct and consistent work on lengthening the spine in particular will create space between the bones. Fluidity and ease of motion result, and the most delicious feeling of well-being— the result of de-compressing the spine and restoring the length the human form was meant to have.

In this book, I hope to communicate to you some accessible and easy-to-implement knowledge about how to pursue flexibility. When you are convinced that something is worthwhile and can enhance your life, you are more likely to undertake it.

What does your body need—stress reduction, pain relief, athletic enhancement? You can take some significant steps on the road to your aims by consulting the book in your hands.

Flexibility training is a versatile tool. It has the power to open the door to a wonderful new world of knowledge and enjoyment of your body's amazing capabilities. You can use this knowledge to cooperate with your body as you create health and fitness. Remember that your body wants to give you what you want. All you have to do is develop a language of communication with it, so you and your body become a team, a smoothly working partnership. You and your fabulous body can accomplish together what you most want to do in your life.

Flexibility training can be an amazing adventure of self-discovery. My wish is that you will find it endlessly rewarding.

Let's begin.

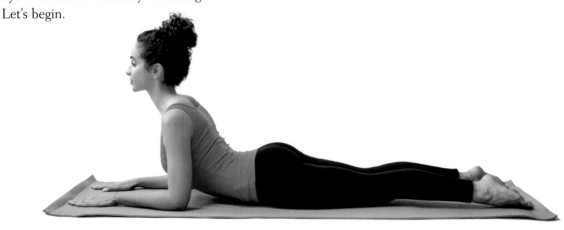

How muscles stretch

What happens inside the muscle:
the "docking" theory

What changes occur in our muscles when we do what we call stretching? We experience a felt *stretch* we identify as pull or tension. Sometimes a good feeling, sometimes uncomfortable, sometimes bordering on pain—there is no other feeling like stretch, and so we always know when it's happening on the outside.

The inside story of a stretch is vastly complex, and shows yet another side of the amazing bodies we have. However, it does make for very dry reading—in fact, it's suspiciously like studying. The sketch presented here is simplified, but it gives you something to visualize when you think about muscles lengthening. Some of us learn best with a visual. (I promise a minimum of technical terms.)

The components of a muscle go from large to small:

MUSCLE → FASCICULUS → FIBER → MYOFIBRIL → SARCOMERE

You just have to remember the *sarcomere*—it's where the stretching action is. By the time we get to the sarcomere, we are down to the microscopic level.

Sarcomeres contain rows of alternating and interlaced *myofilaments* (yet smaller units) called *actin* and *myosin*. You can think of actin as the rowboat and myosin as the dock.

When a muscle contracts, the actin and myosin strands slide over each other and come closer together. The slack between them is taken up. You can say that the rowboats (actin) pull into the docks (myosin). Result: your muscle shortens as you do a resistance exercise.

When you stretch a muscle, the opposite happens. The rowboats (actin) pull away from the docks (myosin). They can pull so far away from each other that each sarcomere can lengthen to 50 per cent beyond its relaxed length. Result: your muscle lengthens as you do a stretch.

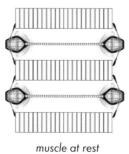

muscle at rest

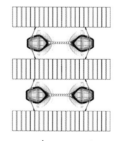

muscle contracting

In addition to the amazing increase in length each sarcomere is capable of reaching, if you systematically stretch your muscles, new sarcomeres actually appear. With more sarcomeres—each of which can lengthen up to 50 per cent beyond its relaxed length—muscles can stretch even more. They just get longer and longer.

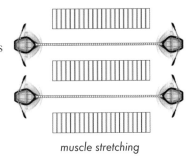

muscle stretching

All around the muscle: the fascial web

This text focuses on the language of muscles in relation to stretching, but a crucial factor also influencing flexibility is connective tissue. This is a brief introduction only, but connective tissue makes up perhaps 30 per cent of muscle mass so, when you stretch muscles, you are also stretching connective tissue.

What fascia is and what it does

There is a web of connective tissue in your body. It surrounds not only your muscles, but your bones, joints, organs—and everything else. It gives your body structure, support, and protection. Referred to as *fascia*, it is all-pervasive in your body. It can help to visualize this web of fascia as a fabric woven of threads, or like the mesh of a fish net with unlimited ability to adapt and change.

It has several layers. The superficial fascia is right under your skin. The deep fascia helps muscles to move, working in partnership with them. This fascial web of tissue wraps right around the muscle, and around every subdivision of the muscle—all the way down to the sarcomere. The muscles and their fascia can be collectively called *myofascia*, and this structure is most relevant in the context of stretching. But all the connective tissue of the fascial network is involved with flexibility. You stretch the whole fascial net when you stretch your muscles.

Connective tissue—quick-change stuff

The cells of the fascial web swim in a material called the extra-cellular matrix, or ECM, consisting of collagen, elastin, and water. Collagen is a strong material, good at resisting forces. Tissues that have more collagen, like tendons, are not easily stretched. Elastin stretches more easily. Tissues containing more elastin give more easily when pulled, like ligaments. And the presence of water (60 to 70 per cent) is what allows you to fall down without injuring yourself—if you're properly hydrated.

This mix of ingredients allows the fascia to change quickly when its composition shifts. If fluid accumulates in the ECM, you may experience swelling and pain. When fluids migrate out because of dehydration, you may feel tight and sluggish.

The ECM also has the property of *viscoelasticity*. This means it's more like a liquid when it's warmer, and more like a solid when it's cooler. Your body temperature affects the consistency of the fascia. When you first get up in the morning your movements are more sluggish, because the fascia is cooler and more solid, which makes it harder to move. After you warm up before your workout you feel more limber, because the fascia has become warmer and more liquid. And after vigorous activity, the fascia is even more liquid, and that is why this post-workout time is optimal for getting your connective tissue and muscles to lengthen while the fascia is still warm, liquid-like, and easily adaptable.

The more you stretch, the more balanced you make the composition of the fascia, with the right proportion of water, collagen, and elastin to keep you more flexible and less stiff. The connective tissue system is the place to go to maximize your flexibility potential.

The body's response to stress and strain

What makes the fascia stiffer and lose flexibility is the body's tendency to deposit more collagen in its ingredient mix. What makes that happen?

We are subjected to all kinds of forces—inside and outside—on a continuing, daily basis. These forces bear on you whether you sit at a desk all day or whether you play a sport at a high level. Your fascia helps you to deal with these forces—gravity among them—and remain in balance. When the fascia develops imbalance—compensation patterns—and the forces become too much for your body, that's when injury results.

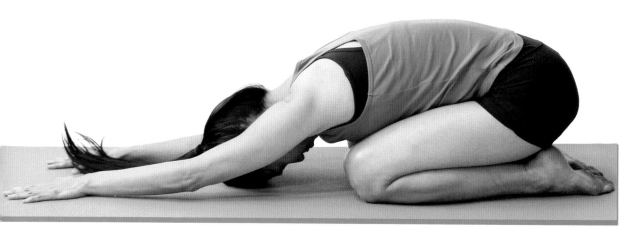

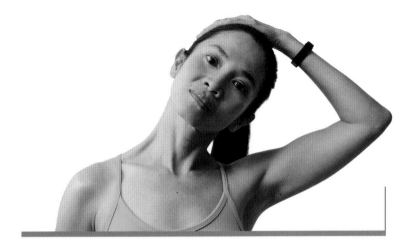

When your body experiences constant or repetitive stress—sitting for a long time, swinging a racquet for hours—it tries to strengthen the parts of your body that are struggling under unequal forces. Its answer to the situation is always the same: it thickens the fascia by putting down more collagen in those stressed spots. More collagen means less elastin and water. And, since collagen resists stretching and there is now more of it in the fascia, you experience a net loss of flexibility—and feel stiffer—when the balance of fascia composition shifts toward collagen and away from elastin and water.

You can remedy this situation by consistent stretching. By pulling your muscles—and fascial web—into length again, you counteract the stiffening effects of collagen, and encourage the body to adjust the fluid balance of your connective tissue more toward the perfect mix.

THE MELT METHOD®

This is a very effective tool for keeping the superficial fascia of your connective tissue well hydrated, and works very well with a flexibility practice. See *Further Study: Flexibility Resources* on p. 185 for more information.

New world of stretching

The fascia is organized in directional lines throughout the body. Efficient ways of stretching are developing that pay attention to these fascial lines, and are able to address tightness and pain all the way down the track. (*Stretch to Win*, by Ann and Chris Frederick, sets forth one of these new systems. The authors integrate fascia with muscles in their flexibility protocols.) In this text, we reference the muscular system to discuss stretching, but we offer this brief discussion of the connective tissue to give you greater awareness of the wider implications of your flexibility practice—you are not just stretching muscles, but the entire fascial web that surrounds and invests them.

There is so much to say about fascia; this section is the merest scratch of the surface.

How muscles respond to stretching

Here are a few strategies that respect the characteristic ways your body behaves when it stretches:

- **Stretching each side separately will yield greater range than stretching both sides at once.** You can see this when you do a simple test. Perform the quadriceps stretch 49 (see p. 106) with both legs; then stretch each leg separately. You will probably be able to pull your heel closer to your buttocks when you stretch one leg at a time. Also, when you do a stretch that involves using your body weight, such as stretch 55 (see p. 115) for your calves, if you drop just one heel off the surface you can shift all your weight over to that side. If you drop both heels off the surface at once, you must distribute your weight between both heels.

- **Stretch the less flexible side first.** Your body tends to give its best effort to the first thing you do. If you know that your left hamstring is less flexible than your right, stretch the left one first. After you do the right side, you can return to the left for some extra time. This will help even out your flexibility range.

- **The body responds with more range of motion when stretches are repeated more than once.** The body is learning what you want it to do, how to become a good partner for your mind as you create your flexible body. It needs a little time to get used to a position, and you will often find that, after a little rest, your body will open up more the second time you do the stretch.

- **Neutralize the stretch reflex.** Whenever a muscle is stretched, its response is to contract. This is why ballistic stretching (see box on p. 32) is not recommended— because that's exactly what happens when you stretch by vigorously bouncing. When you stretch to increase range of motion, (a) begin with a completely relaxed muscle; and (b) stretch slowly, taking your time (see *Longer Static Stretching*, p. 33). This will keep the stretch reflex from occurring, and help you achieve a much greater range of motion in the stretched muscles.

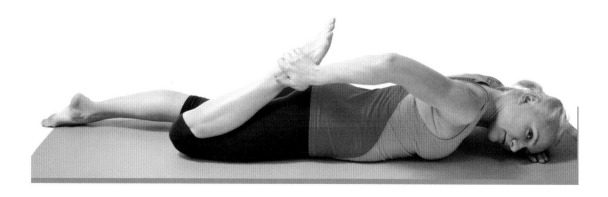

Make stretching work for you: tailored to fit

What makes you *you*? In the whole world, there is only one person with precisely your combination of qualities—you. And that is why the stretching program you carefully craft yourself will be a perfect fit.

Some relevant aspects of your makeup are the activities you do, the physical challenges you face, the goals you have, your emotional outlook, your mental set.

This section offers some concepts to think about as you construct a stretching plan that is uniquely your own. All humans are similar to each other in many ways. That is why there is any basis at all for disseminating information that can possibly help a set of people. But when you get down to the nitty gritty of building a flexibility program, remember that you are the only person on the planet who possesses your particular package of traits. Flexibility is not a one-size-fits-all undertaking. There are some decisions to make. You have the final responsibility—and the wonderful pleasure—of putting together your personal-best stretching line-up.

As you begin developing a stretching strategy that fits you, consider the building blocks below:

Explore other sections of this book

Here is an abundance of solutions and choices to help make assembling your customized flexibility program an easy thing.

From Part One: before you stretch

See what suggestions presented in the remaining sections of *Part One* appeal to you. *Ways to Stretch* (see p. 31) describes a selection of stretching methods to use when you practice flexibility. *Using the Tool of Breathing* (see p. 34) adds an additional layer of variety. *What Muscles to Stretch* (see p. 36) gives you some criteria for choosing priority body areas as your focus. And *When to Stretch* (see p. 40) completes the picture with designs for inserting a stretching session into appropriate slots in your schedule.

From Part Two: your stretch repertory

Consult this section for your complete repertory of stretching techniques, with detailed instructions on how to practice each one, plus photographs and muscle illustrations. As you read the text and look at the pictures, thoughts about how you can use these stretches will occur to you. They will probably be good ideas that fit you well—take a few notes.

From Part Three: stretch sequences

This section covers many situations in which stretching can be your friend. Take some time to browse through and mull over them. *Stretch Before and After Common Physical Activities* (see p. 142) couples various aspects of performing the physical activities discussed with recommended ways to stretch.

From Part Four: your fit and flexible body

The section that can really pull it all together for you is *Create Your Own Stretching Routines* (see p. 174). Having a planned stretching program will help make sure you start one—and stick with it long enough to see some results from your diligence.

It's all about you

This is not usually a positive phrase; it mostly means "other people matter, too—not just you." In this context, though, it's absolutely necessary. Ensuring that your new flexibility program will work for you is a paramount requirement for its success. Stack the deck in your favor with the following information.

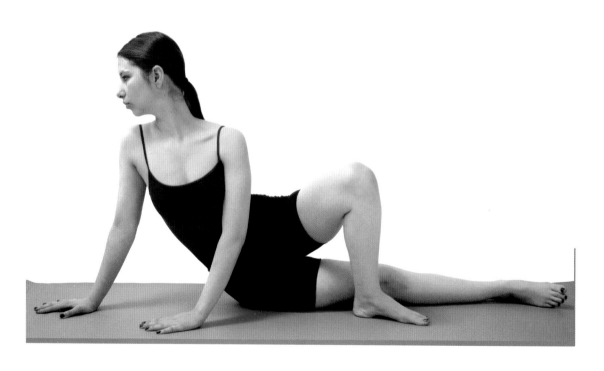

Stretching in a group

If you are new to stretching, taking a class is a good way to get some instruction under your belt before you venture out on your own. Group fitness schedules at gyms and health clubs are likely to include at least a few flexibility classes. When we exercise in a group, it is hard to avoid looking at everyone else in the class. Add to this the competitive atmosphere that prevails in today's fitness climate, and it's easy to become intimidated when you set out to learn a new fitness skill. If your teacher is competent—even inspiring—you will soon be at your ease and focusing on yourself.

When you stretch in a group, remind yourself:

- **Comparing your ability with that of others is irrelevant.** When you see a very flexible person, you have no idea what kind of training his current level of flexibility entailed. Personally, if I'm jealous of someone else's ability, it always helps when I tell myself: if I trade flexibility levels with that person, I will get the rest of his life, too. Do I want that? My answer is invariably "no." You are probably happy with enough facets of your life that you wouldn't want someone else's whole enchilada.

- **Focus on yourself (it's all about you!).** The process of connecting with your body in the stretching moment is so fascinating that you may actually forget to look at the other people in the room.

- **Stretching is not a competition.** Each person moves along his own individual developmental continuum. Wouldn't it be boring if everyone on the planet were the same? We would have nothing to discuss with anyone else.

Some ingredients for your mix

Some components that make people individuals—and influence their stretching progress:

- **How elastic your connective tissues are—in muscles and joints.** The more you stretch, the more elastic these tissues will become.

- **How much tension resides in your muscles.** The signals you send from your mind to your body can release much of this tension.

- **How much strength and coordination you have,** for example, for playing a sport or dancing the ballet.

- **How your bones and joints are structured.** You have the least control over this one. However, unless you are going for extreme stretch—as in a split, or lifting your leg to the side as in ballet—your structure will probably not limit your ability to stretch. If you want to know for sure, a good chiropractor can tell you what's going on.

- **Where your "edge" is.** In a stretch, this is the place where the stretchy feeling threatens to turn into pain. To shift the edge, you add a little more intensity, take away a little—rock the edge. Your edge is in a different spot from someone else's. For example, in stretch 53 (see p. 110), when you reach your edge, your torso may be closer to your thighs than someone else's when he reaches his.

Final reflections

Crucial to your stretching progress is a positive, hopeful attitude. When you embark on a program of flexibility training, you must allow your body time to adapt and improve. The body is a fast learner, but it still needs some time to figure out what on earth you're asking it to do. Changes in your range of motion may start small, but they will accumulate. Your body will respond to your persistence and get the message.

If you hit what seems to be a full stop in your progress, have patience. This may be a plateau, common in sports training. Don't worry. Your body is just gathering information, gearing up for its next forward leap. One way to measure your progress is with a "stretching barometer." Note how far you can go into a stretch—like stretch 52 (see p. 109). How far are your hands from the floor when you start? Measure by eye, or you can even measure with a ruler. Keeping tabs on your progress using a barometer encourages you to keep practicing.

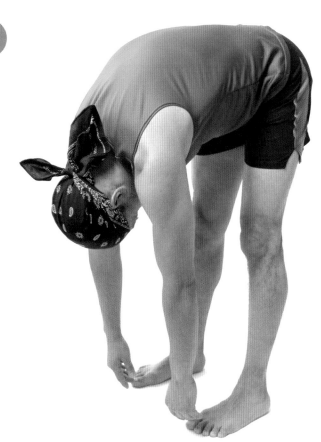

This quote from Dr. Maxwell Maltz's *Psycho-Cybernetics* gives you some inkling of your potential power to advance and improve:

> *The "self-image" sets the boundaries of individual accomplishment. It defines what you can and cannot do. Expand the self-image and you expand the "area of the possible.*[3]

Your ideal flexibility plan will emerge. Do some trials—make some errors. It's all good.

Ways to stretch: how to do it

Types of stretching

Books on stretching classify stretching methods according to different rules. Some authors classify Static Stretching as a separate type from Passive Stretching. There are other subgroups like Passive/Active and Active-Assisted. I prefer a simpler division: Active Stretching and Passive Stretching, with variations on those two main types.

Active stretching

In this method, the muscles opposing the ones stretching are contracting. Example: a front kick, executed with your own muscular power—and then held at the highest point of the kick. The hamstrings (back of the leg) are stretching; the quadriceps (front of the leg) are contracting.

Active Stretching is important for arts and disciplines like ballet and gymnastics. They require the athlete to hold limbs and torso in stationary positions, which are also stretched positions. This book does not discuss this type of Active Stretching. It's mentioned here to show you that flexibility study is a wide world.

Stretch in Motion and PNF Stretching (both discussed below) use components of Active Stretching, but these do not really fit the strict definition above, since the muscles stretching are the same ones that contract (contract and relax in sequence).

Passive stretching

This basically means that your muscles are not contracting; instead, you do everything you can to get them to relax. Their stretch comes from an outside force. That force can be a trainer or partner assisting with the stretch; a prop such as a towel or wall; or you can supply the force yourself in various ways, such as leaning forward or pulling one body part with another (for example, pulling the fingers of one hand with the other).

This book concentrates on methods of Passive Stretching.

Your stretching method catalogue

Passive Stretching protocols can be classified as some variation of:

1   Moving into and out of a stretch.
2   Holding a stretch position.
3   Using resistance at some point during a stretch.

This section gives you a lexicon of methods that have worked for me, both personally and in my teaching practice.

BALLISTIC STRETCHING

Ballistic Stretching is an older method, now pretty much out of favor. It involves vigorous bouncing in and out of the stretch, which is generally considered to activate the body's "stretch reflex": because of the violence of the movement, the body immediately contracts the muscle you just stretched, and your net flexibility gain is zero.

Moving into and out of a stretch

- **Stretch in Motion.** Here you move into a stretch, then out of it, in rhythm. This does not imply any bouncing, but uses a lift-then-lengthen technique instead.

  Example: To stretch your calf using Stretch in Motion, stand in a split stance—one leg in front, knee bent, and one behind, leg straight (see stretch 54a, p. 112). Come up onto the ball of your back foot, then reach your heel down to the floor. Continue this rhythmic up-and-down motion for two sets of eight repetitions. Repeat with the other leg.

  A common term in use today for this way of stretching is *dynamic* stretching.

- **Rhythmic Breathing.** This is a much slower method of moving into and out of a stretch. On a long, slow exhale, move deeper into the stretch position. On the inhale, decrease the pressure. This doesn't mean you pull out of the stretch—just let up slightly on the intensity. (See also *Using the Tool of Breathing*, p. 34.)

  Example: To stretch your lower back using Rhythmic Breathing, lie on the floor on your back, knees to your chest, with one hand on each knee (see stretch 11a, p. 59). On a long, slow exhale, pull your knees farther in toward your chest; feel your lower back stretch. On the inhale, decrease the strength of your pull, and feel the stretch lessen slightly.

Holding a stretch

I use two variations of this technique: Shorter Static Stretching and Longer Static Stretching. They differ only in the length of time you hold the stretch. Enter the stretch you have chosen; align your body as optimally as you can. Hold the position. Locate the stretchy feeling with your mind. When you feel your body's resistance diminish, move a little farther into the stretch.

- **Shorter Static Stretching.** Hold the stretch for 30 to 45 seconds.

- **Longer Static Stretching.** Hold the stretch for one minute or longer. Depending on your goal and flexibility level, three or four minutes is not unfeasible.

  Example: To stretch your buttocks using Shorter Static Stretching, sit on a chair with your right foot on the floor and your left ankle crossed over your right knee (see stretch 38, p. 94). Lift your sacrum and lower back up and out of your hips, begin to lean slowly forward, and keep your back flat. Concentrate on the felt stretch; keep a steady pressure. Hold for 30 to 45 seconds. Repeat on the other side.

Using resistance during a stretch

- **PNF Stretching.** "PNF" stands for Proprioceptive Neuromuscular Facilitation. There are a couple of variations on this technique. I use the following one:

  Place your body in the stretch position you have chosen. Contract the muscle you are stretching as hard as you can—really access it—for a specified length of time. Hold the contraction for eight slow counts, four counts, two—develop your own practice protocol.

  Here is the trick: when your chosen count is complete, relax the muscular contraction, and *immediately* move a little farther into the stretch position. This does not mean release the *position*—relax the *contraction*. There is a split second between the moment you release the contraction and the muscle's relapse into its former degree of stiffness. If you seize that instant—before the body starts thinking, "Oh, I remember: I'm tight here"—you will gain a quite remarkable increase in range in that muscle. But you must *not* delay, or you will lose that tiny window of possibility.

  This is an intense technique. Repeat several times, designing your own hold variations, depending on how your body feels about doing it.

  Example: To stretch your hamstrings using PNF Stretching, stand on your left leg and place your straight right leg onto a chair or a table (see stretch 53, p. 110). Lift your back straight up and away from your legs; lean slowly forward; and keep your back flat. Push your leg down against the surface as hard as you can—the hamstring muscles in the back of your leg will activate. Hold for your chosen count. At the moment you relax the hamstring contraction, see how much farther forward you can lean your flat-back torso into the stretch position. After your chosen number of repetitions, repeat on the other side.

REMEMBER

The goal you have in mind determines the character and duration of the stretch you do. See *Part Four: Create Your Own Stretching Routines* (p. 174) for more on this.

Note: Not every stretching method is suitable for every stretch. A good instructor can help you match the protocol with the stretch, and also your own body awareness—which will develop as you practice flexibility.

Using the tool of breathing

Breathing: open the door to flexibility

The passage of oxygen in and out of our lungs is what we call "breathing." Thousands of times a day, every day of our lives, this process goes on. When we want to say that something is part of the fabric of our lives, we say it is "as natural as breathing." Since breathing goes on non-stop, we are not always aware of it, tending to take it for granted. Yet, consider how vital breathing is to our existence. We can live three weeks without food, three days without water, but only three minutes without air (15 minutes at the very outside before brain death).

Breathing is a semi-conscious process, which means we have some control over its tempo. Faster breathing signals the body to be on the alert; slower breathing calms it down. This becomes important as we seek to relax and open the body through stretching. If we gasp, or hold our breath, the body goes into survival-alert mode. We have all experienced the involuntary intake of breath triggered by an unexpected event. We are hard-wired this way, because survival is our body's first priority. Holding our breath is similar. The body knows its breath-holding limit (30 seconds for the average untrained person), and the clock starts ticking as soon as we forget to exhale. This is not conducive to relaxation. The body has other things on its mind.

The bottom line is: if we want to profit maximally from stretching, we must coax our body to relax. We must convince our body that it is in a safe place, that it is okay for it to let tension go. Correct, conscious stretching is capable of releasing deeply held, tight areas in the body—of which we may not even be aware until we feel and release them. But if we don't breathe deeply and slowly, the body just will not open. Breathing is your ticket to stretching success.

How to use it

For most methods of stretching, paying attention to breathing slowly and deeply, without gasping or holding the breath, is sufficient. Spend a few moments noticing how you breathe naturally. Do you lift your shoulders when you breathe? Do you expand your abdomen as well as your chest when you breathe? Or do you not expand anywhere at all?

See if you can take a good, full breath that widens your ribcage without lifting your shoulders. Your chest will also deepen a little. Once you experience ribcage and chest expansion, see if you can add abdominal relaxation and increase its space as well. On the exhale, the ribcage and chest deflate again, and you can contract your abdomen slightly as the breath leaves that area.

It might be a good idea to take a few minutes before your stretch practice to familiarize your body with this enhanced way of breathing. In the thick of your session, especially when you are learning new techniques, you may forget to breathe like this. But, as repetition makes the concepts and movements more familiar to you, it will be easier to hold more than one thing in your mind.

This basic, heightened-breathing method is appropriate for the following stretching techniques:

- Shorter Static Stretching.

- Longer Static Stretching.

- PNF Stretching (see p. 33).

Stretch in Motion

This method presents a slightly different case. You will likely be using Stretch in Motion as part of a warm-up to prepare your body for a vigorous activity, so your breathing tempo will naturally increase. Just keep your shoulders relaxed as you let the breath flow in and out.

Rhythmic Breathing

The case of Rhythmic Breathing (see p. 32) is somewhat different again. Here you move more deeply into the stretch on your long, slow exhale, and relax the intensity of your position on the inhale. By joining a very slight motion with the timing of your breathing, and adding concentration, you can tune in to the smallest variations in muscular feeling. By mentally "cocking an ear" to your body's reactions as you hold the stretch, you can respond instantly—a little more pressure, a little less. You can feel tiny changes in your body's tension and relaxation levels. It is possible to merge so completely with your body that you approach a meditative state.

In terms of inducing your body to relax, Rhythmic Breathing is a star in your arsenal of tools. What it really does is trick your body into sinking more deeply into a stretch. From your body's point of view, it knows you are going to ask for an intense stretch during one exhale only. Then it will get a break when you inhale and slightly release the pressure. So it will likely go there for you. However, note the degree of stretch your muscles have before you do this technique and check again afterwards. Probably you have sneakily wheedled your body into increasing its range—behind its back, as it were.

You might want to plan a certain number of breaths to complete during a particular stretch. For example, try ten breaths and see what results you get.

What muscles to stretch: matching flexibility to activity

How to choose

We know that flexibility is specific to each muscle group around a joint (see *Introduction*, p. 9). In fact, it is not only specific to each joint, but to each movement within a joint.

What does this mean? Take hamstring flexibility. When you stretch by standing on one leg and placing the other straight leg up on a surface (see stretch 53, p. 110), there are several ways to point your toes:

- Straight up toward the ceiling.

- Toward the midline of your body.

- Away from the midline of your body. (And variations in between.)

The range of motion in your hamstring (torso bent forward, leg straight) may not be equal in each of these toe positions.

So, we all should stretch every muscle we can get our hands on, at every possible joint angle. On a regular basis. That would be the ideal thing. Hmmm.

I mention this to give you an idea of how large is the concept of having a flexible body.

Practically speaking, though, given the schedules of life, there may be some time limits on our flexibility sessions. So, here are some guidelines for efficient directions you can take as you pick muscles you want to concentrate on in your stretching practice.

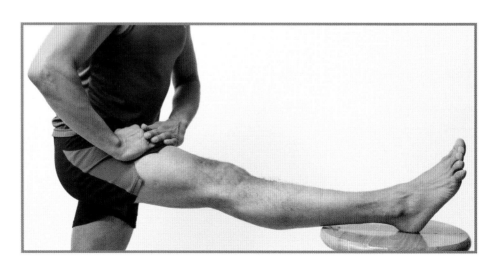

First things first: definitely, everybody stretch your spine!

Attaining and maintaining a mobile spine is of paramount importance to your mobility. Your spine is an amazing, multi-movement structure, and you want to keep it that way. Because of the arrangement of its many bones, it has a large native repertory of movements: it can flex forward, extend upwards and back, extend laterally to both sides, and rotate to both sides. To a large extent, the condition of your spine determines your biological age (see *Introduction*, p. 9, and *Supporting Flexibility*, p. 178). Take a good look at people who are not able to bend and turn easily. The spinal stiffness you observe is largely what makes you perceive them as "old." Staying young—and being perceived that way—is largely a function of a "youthful" spine: flexible, easily movable without a second thought.

A good body-awareness goal is developing the feeling of each vertebra moving independently. Feel stretch all the way along your spine. When you do the Spinal Roll-Down and Roll-Up (see *Moving Warm-Ups*, p. 136), imagine each bone in the vertebral chain as a single pearl on a whole strand of them. Two helpful techniques for creating this feeling are stretches 15 and 16 (see pp. 66 and 67). For well-rounded spine flexibility, try out all the stretches in the *Back* section and see which ones help you most.

Clues elsewhere in this book

Many sections of this book necessarily dovetail and overlap. Look for ideas about which muscles to stretch in *When to Stretch* (see p. 34), and in all the sections of *Part Three: Stretch Sequences* (see p. 134). Take an inventory of how your body feels, or think about what you're planning to do in the way of physical activity. Here is a summary of the complete discussions you'll find in *Part Three*.

Stretch before and after common physical activities (see p. 142)

- Basketball
- Cycling
- Racquetball and handball
- Running
- Swimming
- Walking
- Yoga

Stretch throughout your day (see p. 156)

- Upon waking in the morning
- Using the computer
- Prolonged sitting
- Driving
- Before going to sleep

Stretch to relieve common areas of pain (see p. 161)

- Neck and shoulder
- Lower back and sacrum
- Hip
- Knee

Stretch to increase range of motion (see p. 167)

- Neck
- Shoulder
- Hamstring/lower-back connection
- Hip flexors/quadriceps

Note: When you want to relieve pain or stiffness, stretch not only in the area of actual soreness, but also look at areas distant from the site of discomfort. For example, stretching your upper back may eliminate lower-back discomfort.

How much muscle range do you need?

Once you decide which muscles to stretch, think about what goal you want to set for their flexibility. What range do they need to have? As you have already read (see *Introduction*, p. 9), determine your flexibility goal according to the activity you want to be mobile enough to do. For example:

For daily life: you need enough flexibility to bend down and pick up something you dropped on the floor.

For aerobic dance: you need enough flexibility to lift your knee to 90 degrees without tucking your pelvis under.

For gymnastics: you need enough flexibility to execute a split.

Figure out the range you need in a couple of ways:

- **For a life action, through your own observation:** to see over my shoulder, I must be able to turn my head a little farther.

- **For a new skill, from information given by a skilled instructor:** to execute a back bend well, my shoulders must be open enough to allow me to straighten my arms.

The flexibility reserve. In their book *Stretch to Win*, Ann and Chris Frederick speak about the "flexibility reserve." Through their experience working with many athletes, they have found that having 20 per cent more flexibility than you need for your activity makes injury much less likely. They help their clients develop this reserve in the trunk, spine, shoulders, pelvis, and hips.

Extra flexibility helps you:

- If you fall and land in an awkward position. Your body tissues can handle being suddenly forced farther than their usual range.

- If you reach a little higher or farther back than normal in the heat of a game. You won't tear a muscle.

- In cold weather, when it's hard to keep your muscles warm. Your extra flexibility saves the day.[4]

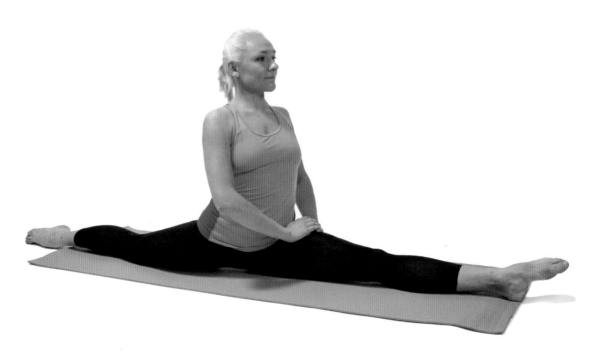

When to stretch: the right timing for your activities and goals

First ...

When should you stretch? The short answer is: any time you feel like doing it. Any time it occurs to you that a good stretch is just the thing. Any time you can feel better combining stretching with something you're doing. Any time stretching can make you feel better after you've done something. Make stretching your go-to feel-better tool. There are no limits on its use.

Examples

Remember that the bodies we inhabit are "moving machines." This is their nature: it's where they live. So, if you haven't moved for a while (for example, a couple of hours), if you are listening, your body will start telling you to get moving. It has no words; instead, you will get feelings like, "my neck feels stiff"; "my shoulders are slumping"; "my hips feel antsy."

You can respond to this get-moving directive with some off-the-cuff, improvisatory stretches. Let your body's feelings dictate the stretches you might use. Even if stretching was Greek to you before you picked up this book, you now have a whole repertory from which to choose (see *Part Two: Your Stretch Repertory*, p. 42). The more familiar with those movements you get, the more they will seep into your subconscious, like water into soil. They will start occurring to you when you feel your body's get-moving signal. For example:

- If your neck feels stiff, where precisely is that feeling? Back, side, front? Pick a stretch from the *Neck* section (see pp. 44–49).

- If your shoulders are slumping, the front muscles will be contracted, and hence shorter. Lengthen them again with a front-shoulder stretch from the *Shoulders and Chest* section (see pp. 50–57).

- If your hips feel antsy, is it your butt, inner thighs, side hip? Go to the *Hips* (see pp. 90–99) or *Thighs* (see pp. 100–110) section and select a position that fits the situation.

Tune in to the feelings you get from your body—which are there, even if you've never paid attention before—and let them steer you in the stretching direction you need at that moment. Your body will be delighted to get such a good answer to its request.

Second ...

The stand-alone stretching session

If you have designated a time during your day to address a flexibility issue you've targeted (see *What Muscles to Stretch*, p. 36), warm up your body generally first (see *Prepare to Stretch*, p. 136). You will get the most mileage out of your scheduled stretching session if your body is already primed with all those pluses you get from warming up.

Before and after physical activities

- **Before.** After a general warm-up (see *Prepare to Stretch*, p. 136), continue getting ready for your activity using Stretch in Motion to prepare the muscles you will be using (see *Ways to Stretch*, p. 31). Your muscles will become limber, and also geared up to work at an intensified level. (See *Prepare to Stretch*, p. 136, for a description of the perfect warm-up that precedes a good aerobic dance class.)

You could experiment with Shorter Static Stretching before an activity, depending on what that activity is (see *Ways to Stretch*, p. 31). For example, your ability to perform the slow, sustained movements of yoga will probably not be affected if you hold a warm-up stretch position for 30 seconds. But for the most part, stay away from static stretching before a vigorous cardiovascular workout. It is a stellar technique for increasing range of motion, but it doesn't make muscles rough and ready.

- **After.** Take advantage of the after-workout state of your muscles: they're warm, tired, less resistant to increasing range of motion—they won't fight you. Your body says, "Whatever. I'm too tired to care." Aha! Pounce on this delicious, euphoric, relaxed muscular state to get some real flexibility gains. Here is where Longer Static Stretching and PNF Stretching really shine (see *Ways to Stretch*, p. 31). (Of course, use general body movements to cool down first.)

There is a full discussion of how to optimize stretching around physical activity in *Part Three: Stretch Before and After Common Physical Activities*, p. 142.

A TIP FROM BALLET

A dear ballet teacher once told me: stretching and jumping are not a good combination. Jumping is ballet's cardiovascular exercise—it is seriously intense work, especially if done correctly and safely. He was saying, in effect, that extreme stretching temporarily weakens muscles. This is an idea supported by today's scientific studies, and my teacher, trained in Russia in the traditional system, was giving me the benefit of 100+ years of Russian ballet experience. His translated advice: to jump, you must be able to access your optimum power, so avoid long stretches before attempting it.

41

PART ONE BEFORE YOU STRETCH

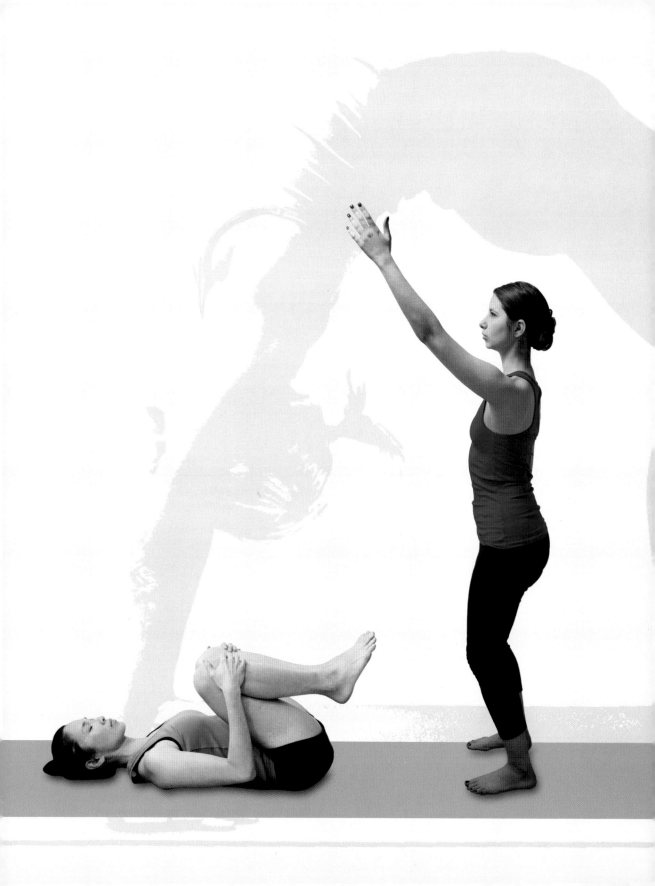

PART TWO
YOUR STRETCH REPERTORY

Delve into the ingredient mix for your stretching program—an organized list of stretches at a glance. Here we get down to brass tacks with the basics. How can you allow your body to release gently into a stretch? How can you align yourself correctly so other body areas do not become stressed? And—crucial to your stretching education—exactly where should you be feeling muscular pull? The instructions emphasize giving your body enough time to settle into a position, without rushing into or out of it. A unique plus: increase your sense of calm and minimize fear by creating a partnership between your mind and your body. You will learn to recruit your mind to address your body's tight spots.

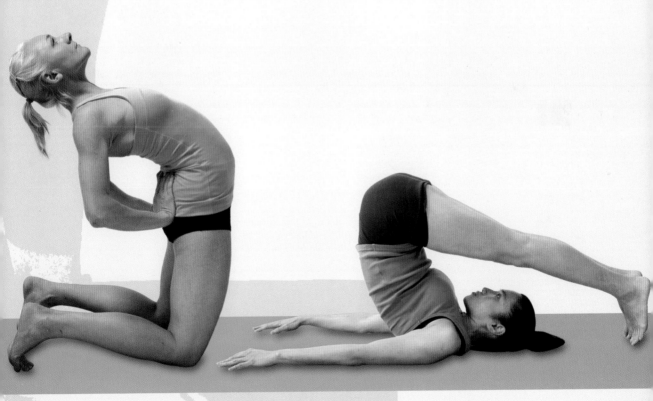

Neck

This section will show you side, back, and front neck stretches. Almost any activity can produce neck stiffness or soreness. Gently lengthen your neck in the area where you feel discomfort.

Causes of stiff neck muscles	• Waking up with a crick in your neck after sleeping in an awkward position. • A long phone conversation in which you hold your head at a constant angle. • Texting—holding your head for 10 minutes at the downward angle many people assume when texting is like having 60 lb (27 kg) of pressure directly on your neck. • Reading—the proper way to hold a book (or e-reader!) to avoid neck stiffness is at eye level. Looking down at a book on your lap stiffens your neck. • Post-sport fatigue—your muscles can stiffen up in response to a playing session involving many head movements.
Causes of sore or aching neck muscles/muscles in spasm	• Carrying heavy bags (such as groceries), which may cause you to hike up your shoulders and constrict your neck. • Any change in habitual head-movement habits that are repeated many times, for example, looking in a different direction because some piece of equipment has been moved to a new spot in your office. • Playing a sport like racquetball, in which rapid head movements are important for tracking the flight of the ball.
Injuries eased by stretching	• Neck muscle strain. • Whiplash (neck sprain)—if mild. • Cervical nerve stretch syndrome (burning sensation radiating down neck and shoulder). • Wry neck (painfully twisted and tilted neck).

Pinpoint the area of discomfort (this connects your mind with your body), and choose the stretch that most closely reaches that spot.

For guidance on stretch duration, see pp. 32–33. To discover how to use breathing to deepen the stretch, see pp. 34–35.

1 neck: side

- **The Setup:** Sit or stand comfortably with spine straight and shoulders relaxed. Release tension from your neck by turning to each side a couple of times.

- **The Stretch:** Reach up with your left hand and pull your head gently to the left side. At the same time, sink your right shoulder down and away from the pull. Your aim is to create length between the right shoulder and the right ear, which you will feel as a steady pull. That is the stretch feeling you're always looking for. Do the stretch on the other side as well.

- **Enhance Your Flexibility:** When you finish this stretch, using whatever breathing technique and duration you have chosen, it can be helpful to take your head—in its side-lying position—between your hands. Lift it gently back up until your ears are parallel to the floor again. If your hands carry the weight of your head, your neck muscles will get a little rest. Doing this will prolong the relaxation effect of the stretch, instead of cancelling it out by forcing the neck muscles to work immediately. Muscles are more likely to retain their new, happy, stretched state if they are not suddenly shocked out of it.

ENLIST YOUR MIND

Cultivate awareness of your neck's state as you move through your day. Create a little checkpoint schedule, and ask yourself at those moments, "Is my neck tense? Can I relax it?" Think: shoulders relaxed and away from neck—create lots of space.

KEY

- Trapezius
- Levator scapulae
- Scalenes
- Sternocleidomastoid

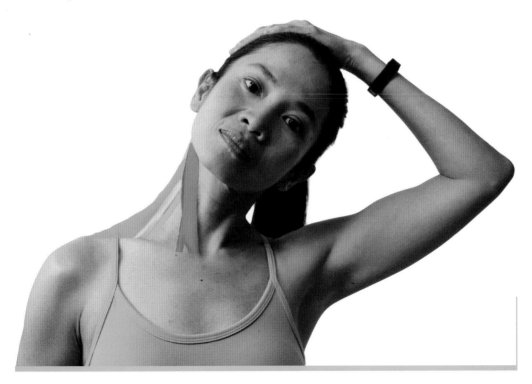

2 neck: back

- **The Setup:** Sit or stand comfortably with spine straight and shoulders relaxed. Locate the little bony nodules at the base of your skull. They are on the left and right sides at the back.

- **The Stretch:** Lift up underneath those spots with several fingers of both hands; let your neck lengthen in response to the lift; and let your head bow forward as your neck lengthens. It's important not to jam your neck vertebrae together. Do this stretch with the idea of creating length in the back of your neck. At the same time, sink your back and shoulders straight down and away from the pull. When you want to release the position, assist your neck muscles as they return your head to its original position by continuing to lift and pull up under your skull.

- **Enhance Your Flexibility:** Keep your shoulders relaxing downward. All stretches use the principle of pulling two fixed points apart. This is what creates length in the muscle. You will be pulling one point down—the shoulder(s)—and the other point up and away from it—the neck.

ENLIST YOUR MIND

If you do this whole group of stretches in sequence, your neck may feel longer when you finish. You may feel you are carrying it higher. You may feel a release of tension. Freeing the neck canal from tension may also reduce your stress level. Any of these results indicate stretching success.

KEY

☐ Splenius cervicis
■ Splenius capitis
☐ Trapezius

Note: In the illustration shown here, some of the neck muscles being stretched overlay the thumb. All muscles shown are stretching on both sides of the body.

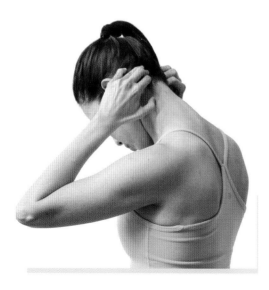

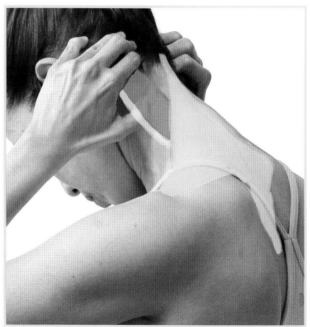

3 neck: back diagonal

- **The Setup:** Sit or stand comfortably with spine straight and shoulders relaxed. As in stretch 2, locate the little bony nodules at the base of your skull.

- **The Stretch:** As in stretch 2, create length in the back of your neck by pulling up under the little bony nodules at the base of your skull. The back of your neck is now stretching. Next, turn your chin slowly to the right. You will feel the stretch shift from the back of your neck to the side back—on the left side. As before, sink your left shoulder down and away from the pull, and locate the stretchy feeling. As in stretch 1, when you are ready to release the position, take the weight off your neck muscles by using your hands to return your head to its original position. Repeat the stretch on the other side.

- **Enhance Your Flexibility:** Experiment with the placement of your assisting hand as you seek to deepen the stretch gently. You may feel more stretch if you use your fingers to lift your head up under the skull bone. Also, check how the stretch is increased when you place your hand farther up on your head, as in the photograph. Remember: the shoulder sinks down and away, while the opposite hand does the pull.

ENLIST YOUR MIND

Remember that no one can get inside your body and feel its feelings except you—only *your* mind connects with the inside of *your* body. Although we speak as though each body feels the same things, we really don't know that. You are the most accurate judge of what your body feels, and the most capable of giving your body an optimal stretching experience.

KEY
- Semispinalis capitis
- Trapezius

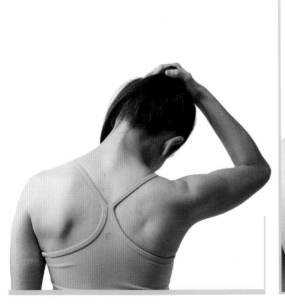
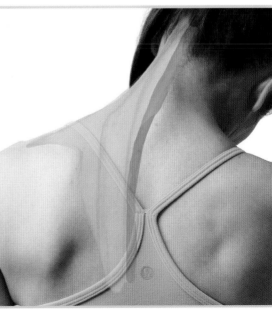

4 neck: front

- **The Setup:** Sit or stand comfortably with spine straight and shoulders relaxed. Begin with the feeling of both shoulders dropping very low, and hold onto this feeling throughout the stretch. It is most important that, in stretching the front of the neck, you do not create constriction in the back of the neck.

- **The Stretch:** Feeling your shoulders dropping down around your ribcage, slowly lift your chin straight up, lengthening your front neck muscles. Locate the pull, and find the highest point that the stretch can reach—beyond that point the back of your neck will begin to constrict. Hold this delicate balance—length in front and length in back—for the duration of the stretch.

- **Enhance Your Flexibility:** Place the tip of your tongue just below your lower teeth (inside your mouth) and press. This increases the stretch, and also contracts the muscles. Your stretch has now become a face exercise as well.

ENLIST YOUR MIND

What does it mean to "locate the stretch"? You can enhance your flexibility training greatly if you build a partnership between your mind and your body. Go through a series of positions with awareness: that is the path to the best results. To get the most for your money, find a way to feel gently into the muscle as you perform each stretch. How you do this will be entirely unique to you. Close your eyes if you like. Here's an idea: identify the difference between how the muscle feels when it's stretching and when it isn't.

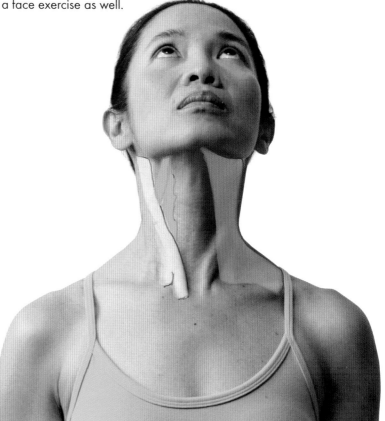

KEY

■ Longus capitis
▢ Sternocleidomastoid
▨ Longus colli
▧ Platysma

Note: All muscles shown are stretching on both sides of the body.

5 neck: front diagonal

- **The Setup:** When you first do this stretch, it may help to stand (or sit) in front of a mirror to get your angles right. But your primary reference will be the stretch you feel. This stretch targets the neck in front, slightly to one side. Make sure your spine is straight, yet relaxed, and your shoulders dropped and at ease.

- **The Stretch:** Lift your chin straight up to the front, so that you feel a pull on the front of your neck as in stretch 4. Hold the balance: lift your chin enough, but not so much that you create shortening in the back of your neck. Slowly turn your lifted chin to the left. The feeling of stretch will shift from the front to the right side of your neck.

    When you want to release the stretch, slowly lower your chin along the line of the lift. Sink your shoulders and let the back of the neck relax, just in case you introduced any strain there during the stretch. Return your dropped chin to the center and continue to let the back of your neck be heavy and relaxed. Repeat the stretch on the other side.

- **Enhance Your Flexibility:** At the peak of the stretch, when your chin is pointed up and to one side, tilt your chin slightly downward toward your shoulder. The stretching intensity will increase.

KEY

Sternocleidomastoid

Longus capitis

Longus colli (vertical)

Platysma

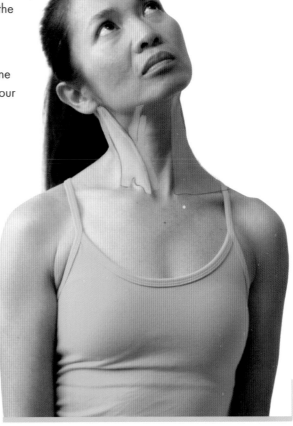

ENLIST YOUR MIND

This is your mantra: sink your shoulders; keep the back of your neck long.

Shoulders and chest

This section discusses stretches for the front and back shoulder, and the chest. Remember that the body is a unified whole, which means muscles stretch in groups, not in isolation. Adjust your position in any stretch to address the area of tightness.

Causes of stiff, sore, or aching shoulder and chest muscles/ muscles in spasm	• Allowing your shoulders to roll forward constantly. • Performing repetitive shoulder movements in an occupation—cashiers, hairdressers, makeup artists. • Playing sports or doing activities that require a lot of shoulder movement—basketball, handball, swimming.
Injuries eased by stretching	• Frozen shoulder. • Rotator cuff tendonitis. • Chest strain.
Additional uses	• Before and after playing sports requiring extensive shoulder movement—basketball, handball, swimming. • Increase shoulder flexibility to the level required for swimming.

Pinpoint the area of discomfort (this connects your mind with your body), and choose the stretch that most closely reaches that spot.

For guidance on stretch duration, see pp. 32–33. To discover how to use breathing to deepen the stretch, see pp. 34–35.

6 front shoulder: elbow bent, using chair

- **The Setup:** Kneel on the floor on all fours (with padding for your knees, if you like) next to a folding chair (or similar—not a cushy armchair!). Place your torso in line with the front edge of the chair. Place your forearm along the front edge of the chair seat, making sure that your elbow is totally supported by the chair—not hanging off the edge. (If your forearm is longer than the chair seat is wide, let your hand/wrist hang over the edge.) Gently press downward with your forearm on the chair seat to make sure that the chair will not tip over under pressure. Adjust your forearm position farther from the chair edge if necessary.

- **The Stretch:** Pressing firmly and gently downward on the chair seat with your forearm, allow your shoulder to sink down between your chest and your upper arm. Your shoulder, armpit, and chest will form an arc whose lowest point will be around your armpit. Feel the stretch in the front of the shoulder (which will be facing downward). The feeling of stretch may extend into your chest. Repeat the stretch on the other side.

- **Enhance Your Flexibility:** Experiment with moving your shoulder slowly backward, and then slowly forward, to find different angles of stretch. The more areas you can bring into play, the more all-around stretch you will gain for your front-of-shoulder area.

ENLIST YOUR MIND

Your mind may take some time to connect the feeling of stretch with the action of the stretch. Once you are fairly certain you have placed your body in the position described left, you may have to forge a new neural pathway for your mind to follow as it catches up with your body. Remember: "neurons that fire together wire together." This is known as Hebb's axiom, coined by Canadian neuropsychologist Donald Hebb in 1949. If you don't immediately feel the stretch, repeat the firing pattern—and you will.

KEY

▮ Anterior deltoid
▮ Pectoralis major

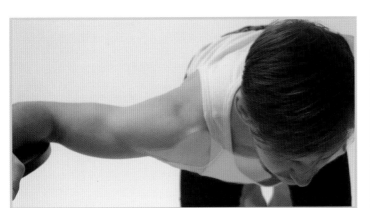

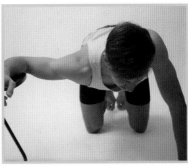

7 front shoulder: arm straight, using doorway

- **The Setup:** Stand facing an open doorway. Stand comfortably with your feet planted solidly underneath you. You should be very well balanced, with your knees slightly relaxed. Extend your right arm straight out to the right. Drop your hand below shoulder level and place your open palm against the edge of the doorway. Monitor your shoulder so that it doesn't hike up; keep it relaxing down, free of tension. Both shoulders should be at the same height.

ENLIST YOUR MIND

Think about making an outward curve in your armpit. Create lots of space in the area between your shoulder and your chest— lots of space to allow further opening as you hold the position. Remember to release all the tension from your neck and relax your knees.

- **The Stretch:** Keeping your arm straight and palm on the doorway edge, slowly turn your torso to the left, away from your extended arm. Look for the feeling of stretch in the front of your right shoulder and/or in your armpit area between shoulder and chest. Repeat with the other arm.

- **Enhance Your Flexibility:** As you continue to concentrate on the feeling of stretch in the front of your shoulder, it will start to open and the feeling of stretch will diminish. Your body is getting used to the degree of flexibility you are requesting from it. If your goal is to gain more range, seize this moment to turn a little more away from your arm and up the intensity of the stretchy feeling. Doing this in small increments will gradually give you more range and freedom in your shoulder.

KEY

▨ Anterior deltoid
▨ Pectoralis major

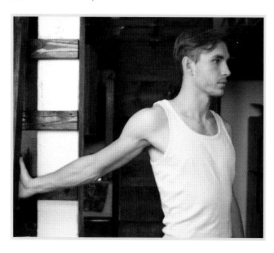
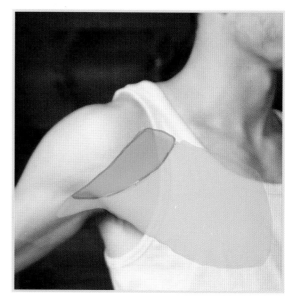

8 back shoulder: standing, using doorway

- **The Setup:** Stand facing an open doorway. Extend your right arm in front of you at shoulder height, with your thumb pointing downward. Grip the edge of the doorway with your right hand. The more secure your grip is, the better: use all four fingers if you can. Place your feet comfortably underneath you, relaxing your knees. You should not feel that you have to balance yourself. Just use a stance width that is normal for you.

- **The Stretch:** Slowly turn your torso into your outstretched arm. Keep your arm straight if you can. The feeling of stretch will appear on the outside of your shoulder as you turn farther into it. Repeat with the other shoulder.

- **Enhance Your Flexibility:** First make sure that you are feeling the stretch in the outside of your shoulder. Then you can experiment with turning farther in the direction of your shoulder. The stretch will travel into your upper back as well.

ENLIST YOUR MIND

Should your mind have trouble connecting to the feeling of stretch, try the other arm first. Sometimes you can feel the stretch more easily on one side. Then you can use that side to teach the other side to feel it as well. Remember that we are not symmetrical in many ways. As you develop the increased connection of your mind with your body using the medium of stretching, you have the power to even out some of the differences between right and left sides, so that they become less disparate.

KEY

◻ Posterior deltoid

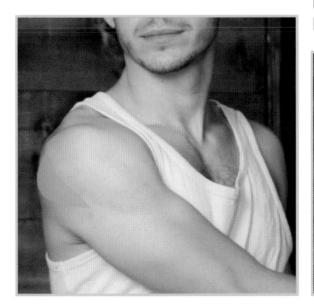

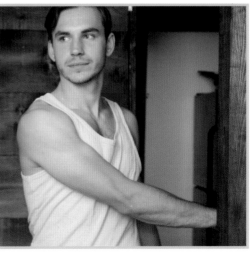

9 back shoulder: squatting, using doorway

- **The Setup:** Stand facing an open doorway (or doorway substitute), a little to the right of center. Extend your left arm in front of you at shoulder height, with your thumb pointing upward. Grip the right edge of the doorway with your left hand. The more secure your grip is, the better: use all four fingers if you can. Place your feet comfortably underneath you, at least shoulder width apart, relaxing your knees.

- **The Stretch:** Bend your knees a little bit more. At the same time, lean backward, away from the doorway, holding on with your left hand. As you bend your knees and lean backward, look for the feeling of stretch on the outside and back of your left shoulder. Repeat the stretch on the other side.

- **Enhance Your Flexibility:** Make sure your butt is not sticking out behind you. Your goal is a comfortably straight torso. Really allow the doorway to support you as you look for the feeling of stretch in the back of your shoulder. Use the support of your core musculature: pull your belly button in to keep your weight off your knees.

ENLIST YOUR MIND

This is a good place to work on the connection between your mind and your stretching body. Bend your knees a little more—see how that affects the intensity of your stretch. Move the position of your arm—a little higher than your shoulder, a little lower. Feel the difference in stretch intensity each position gives you.

KEY
 Posterior deltoid
Rhomboid

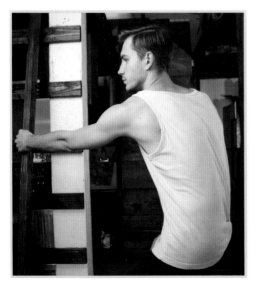

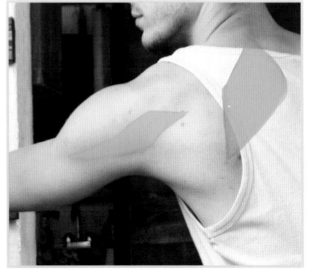

10a chest (breastbone): shoulder-level elbows

The following three stretches will give you a fairly complete opening in your chest area. The different bent-elbow levels allow you to shift the emphasis to higher and lower points of focus. Make sure your doorway or other support won't move when you apply pressure.

- **The Setup:** Stand facing an open doorway. Open your elbows at shoulder height, and place your elbows and forearms against the door frame—one on each side. You should feel supported by the door frame as you lean through it with your shoulders.

  Place one foot behind you and one in front of you. Bend your front knee. Your body should be slightly slanted; it should make a nice line from the top of your head to the heel of your back foot. No sticking your butt out or pushing your pelvis forward. Just relax and let the door frame and the floor support you. Check that the toes of your back foot are placed in front of your heel—not winging out to the side.

- **The Stretch:** Slowly, feeling your way, lean your chest forward. You will feel the stretch in the chest and front-of-shoulder areas.

- **Enhance Your Flexibility:** Adjust your front knee a bit more forward, and feel how that affects the intensity of the stretch. As long as you keep your knee in line with your foot, the knee can go a little in front of the ankle. Make sure your lower-back and sacrum vertebrae are not scrunching together. Keep dropping the shoulders—relax them down around your ribcage.

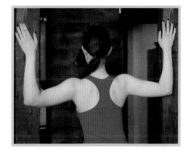

KEY

Pectoralis major (sternal fibers)
Pectoralis minor

Note: All muscles shown are stretching on both sides of the body.

ENLIST YOUR MIND

Stretches are always more effective when your body and mind are partners. At first you will have to make conscious connections, but once your body identifies the place you want to stretch, the connection will occur so quickly you won't notice it happened. In this case, keep thinking: chest through the shoulders, chest forward of shoulders. Push a little with the back foot; adjust the knee slightly forward. Evaluate the effects these thoughts and actions have on your feeling of stretch.

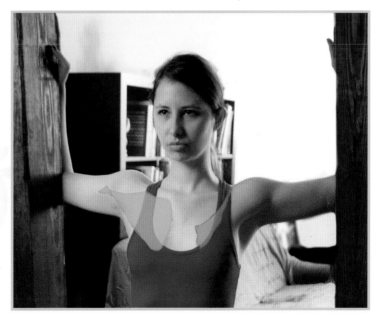

10b chest (collarbone): elbows below shoulder level

ENLIST YOUR MIND

This stretch and the next one, stretch 10c, introduce subtle gradations in the location of the stretchy feeling you get when you do them. You are lowering your elbows, but the stretch is traveling *upward*—to your collarbone area. Look for that feeling. When you practice "looking" for the location of the stretch (of course, we're not really "looking"—more like "searching"), you are forging new neural pathways that unite your mind with what your body is experiencing.

KEY

Pectoralis major (clavicular fibers)

Pectoralis minor

- **The Setup:** Stand facing an open doorway, as in stretch 10a. Open your elbows at shoulder height, and place your elbows and forearms against the door frame—one on each side. Improvise if you need to with whatever stable support you have at home. Your criteria are: (a) stability of support (won't fall over when you lean into it); and (b) correct width to accommodate your elbows (there can be a big difference in elbow span among people).

  One foot goes behind you and one in front. Your front knee is bent. Slant your body to create a nice line from the top of your head to the heel of your back foot.

  Now drop your elbows several inches below shoulder height. This is what's different from stretch 10a—the level of your elbows.

- **The Stretch:** Lean your chest forward as in stretch 10a. You will feel the stretch in the chest and front-of-shoulder areas as before. See if you can feel the stretch shifting to a slightly higher location—more toward your collarbone.

- **Enhance Your Flexibility:** As you continue to push the chest gently through the shoulders, remember to keep your neck long—your chin should not jut out or up, because it will constrict your neck vertebrae. This elbow position carries the stretch upward into your collarbone. If you have any shoulder constriction or stiffness, you may feel some discomfort in the back of your neck. You can remedy this neck/shoulder stiffness by doing extra shoulder stretching. In the meantime, reduce the intensity of your forward push in this stretch, even if it means a temporary lessening of the feeling of stretch in your chest.

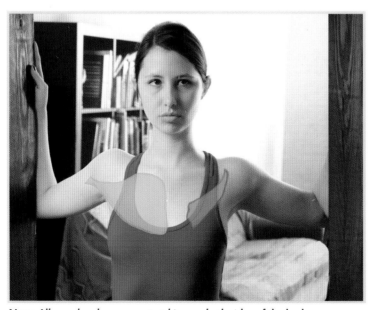

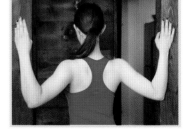

Note: All muscles shown are stretching on both sides of the body.

10c chest (ribcage): elbows above shoulder level

ENLIST YOUR MIND

Practice a check-in with all the elements of good form:

- One straight line from top of head to heel—no butt sticking out.
- Long back of neck to protect neck vertebrae—no chin jutting forward or up.
- Back foot—toes lining up with heel.
- Front knee—in line with toes.
- Shoulders dropped and relaxed.

Once you go through this checklist in your mind a few times—perhaps without even adding the stretch—it will become automatic. From a well-aligned position you can execute any stretch without fear of injury. Plus, when your body is well aligned, every time you stretch, you reinforce your base-line barometer. From this base you can measure your progress as you increase your range of motion.

- **The Setup:** Stand facing an open doorway, as in stretches 10a and 10b. Open your elbows at shoulder height, and place your elbows and forearms against the door frame—one on each side. Improvise with equipment if you need to: use whatever stable support you have at home.

  One foot goes behind you and one in front. Your front knee is bent. Slant your body to create a nice line from the top of your head to the heel of your back foot.

  Lift your elbows several inches above shoulder height. This is the difference between this stretch and stretches 10a and 10b—the level of your elbows.

- **The Stretch:** Lean your chest forward as in stretches 10a and 10b. You will feel the stretch in the chest and front-of-shoulder areas as before. See if you can feel the stretch shifting to a slightly lower location—more toward your ribs.

- **Enhance Your Flexibility:** Here the stretch moves *downward*, into the chest area around your ribs. As you push the chest gently forward through the shoulders, monitor your ribcage to make sure it isn't thrusting forward. This stretch is for your chest—not your ribcage.

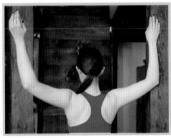

KEY

	Pectoralis major (costal fibers)
	Pectoralis minor

Note: All muscles shown are stretching on both sides of the body.

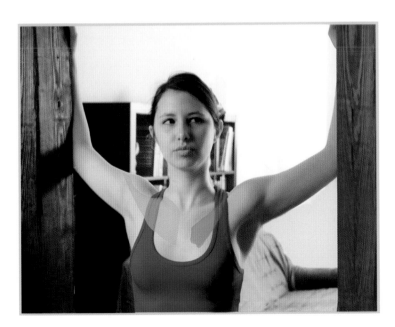

Back

In this section we will cover stretches for the lower and upper back, both in flexion and extension, as well as lengthening moves that encompass the full spine. During each technique, look for the feeling of stretch in the areas described.

Causes of stiff, sore, or aching back muscles/ muscles in spasm	• A whole day of maintaining the upright or sitting position, which compresses spinal discs and pushes the cushioning fluid out from between them. • Sitting at the computer—or any long sitting session, such as attending a business conference. • Playing sports—almost any sport requires constant back use. The examples in this book are basketball, cycling, racquetball/handball, running, swimming, walking, and yoga (see *Stretch Before and After Common Physical Activities*, p. 142). • Any intense or prolonged exercise.
Injuries eased by stretching	• Upper- or lower-back muscle strain (choose appropriate stretch). • Upper- or lower-back ligament sprain (mild) (choose appropriate stretch). • Abdominal muscle strain (obliques, stretch 23).
Additional uses	• Before and after playing sports requiring constant or intense back movement, including twisting movements—basketball, cycling, racquetball/handball, running, swimming, walking. • When you wake up still tired with a nagging backache. Your muscles may be too stiff to allow spine decompression as you sleep.

Pinpoint the area of discomfort (this connects your mind with your body), and choose the stretch that most closely reaches that spot.

For guidance on stretch duration, see pp. 32–33. To discover how to use breathing to deepen the stretch, see pp. 34–35.

PELVIC TUCK AND TILT: WHAT'S THE DIFFERENCE?

What is the difference? Lie on your back on the floor, knees bent and feet on the floor. **Tuck your pelvis:** flatten your lower-back curve against the floor. There will be no space between you and the floor all along your back, and your pubic bone will lift up toward your chest. **Tilt your pelvis:** push your pubic bone down and away from you, and feel that your butt is sticking out. The curve in your lower back returns, and gets bigger. (Keep your ribs on the floor, so that only the pelvis moves.) Now relax everything, and you are in pelvic neutral—neither tucked nor tilted.

11a lower back (flexion): knees to chest

These three stretches are a progression from least intense to most intense. If you are in pain or just beginning your flexibility training, you would probably start with stretch 11a. As your back feels better or you gain more flexibility, you can move to 11b. Stretch 11c, The Plough, requires the most flexibility. In my own case, there was a long summer when I practiced it almost every morning. At the end of the summer I achieved the plough. Moral? With stretching, patience in practice pays off.

- **The Setup:** Lie on a comfortable but supportive surface, such as a carpet or an exercise mat. A bed doesn't provide enough support for your body, although you can wake yourself up with modified versions of some stretches before getting out of bed in the morning (see *Upon Waking in the Morning*, p. 156).

  Make sure the back of your neck is nice and long. This means your chin will be more tucked into your chest than pointed to the ceiling. Cultivate the feeling that some friendly hand is pulling the base of your skull gently along the floor, allowing a long, free feeling to appear in the back of your neck.

- **The Stretch:** Place one hand on each knee (or behind each thigh) and pull your knees toward your chest. Look for a feeling of length in the muscles of your spine below your waist—your sacrum.

- **Enhance Your Flexibility:** Feel how the stretch changes as you alternately slowly sink your butt to the floor and allow it to rise again slightly—without moving your knees. This is good movement education for your sacral muscles.

Note: These muscles lie underneath the arm but, for the purposes of illustration, the muscles are shown overlaying the arm. All muscles shown are stretching on both sides of the body.

ENLIST YOUR MIND

As you pull your knees into your chest, allow your body to become very heavy and really sink into the floor. Neck longer, back so heavy it even goes *through* the floor. Even though you are stretching your lower back/sacral area, allowing other muscles to release contractions you may not be aware of can increase your general relaxation.

KEY

Erector spinae:

- Iliocostalis
- Longissimus cervicis, thoracis
- Spinalis thoracis

- Multifidi

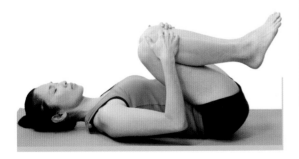

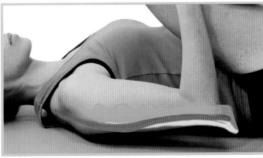

11b lower back (flexion): lower legs extended

- **The Setup:** Lie on your back on a comfortable—but not-too-soft—surface. Keep your neck long and supple, with your chin not quite tucked—but definitely not pointing toward the ceiling.

- **The Stretch:** Begin by pulling your knees gently into your chest. Either use one hand on each knee, or one hand behind each thigh—whichever position is more comfortable for you. (This is the 11a position.) It is okay to allow your butt to lift slightly off the floor.

  Placing one hand on each calf, begin to unfold your lower legs. With your knees still bent, pull the calves toward you. This will make your thighs come closer to your chest, exerting a more intense pull on your lower-back/sacrum area. As you become more flexible, you will be able to adjust your hands on your calves to the position that will give you the greatest degree of possible stretch.

- **Enhance Your Flexibility:** Stretching on your back with the knees bent emphasizes the lower-back/sacrum stretch, with minimum involvement of the backs of your legs (hamstrings). Pay attention to how this variation increases the stretchy feeling (intensity) compared to 11a.

ENLIST YOUR MIND

A clear mental concept always helps your stretching progress. Sure knowledge of what and where the sacrum and lower back actually are will serve you much better than vague ideas about their location. This is particularly important because the back is behind you. Human orientation is naturally focused toward the front, so what's in back is more challenging for us to sense. It is possible to delve into fine detail on this point but, simply put, your lower back is in the area of your waistline. Your belly button is opposite your lumbar (lower-back) vertebrae—in the range of L3 to L5. The sacrum is below that—basically the pelvic area.

Note: In stretches 11b and 11c, the muscles lie underneath the arm but, for the purposes of illustration, the muscles are shown overlaying the arm. All muscles shown are stretching on both sides of the body.

KEY

Erector spinae:

Iliocostalis

Longissimus cervicis, thoracis

Spinalis thoracis

Multifidi

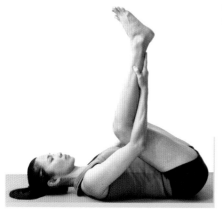

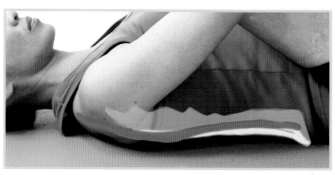

11c lower back (flexion): legs over head

- **The Setup:** As in stretches 11a and 11b, lie on your back on a supportive and comfortable surface. Your neck is long, your chin sinking slightly toward your chest.

- **The Stretch:** There are several ways to enter this stretch, also known as "the plough," which we will explore later (see *Compound Stretches*, p. 124). Here, since this is the most intense of our lower-back/sacrum flexion series, begin as in 11a by pulling your knees gently into your chest, using your preferred hand position—on your knee or behind your thigh. Intensify the stretch by passing through 11b: unfold your lower legs and gently press your thighs toward your chest.

  An optimally executed 11c stretch is close to your maximum lower-back flexion range. You may take many incremental steps on your way to this goal.

  Begin to move into 11c from 11b by giving your butt a push to lift it and take it backward. If you don't need to push with your arms, use your core to bring your bent legs up and over your head. Slowly straighten your legs. The stretchy feeling will increase simultaneously in the backs of your legs and in your lower-back/sacrum area. Hold for your chosen duration; then slowly bend your knees again and return, through stretch 11b, to your original position with knees to chest.

- **Enhance Your Flexibility:** Once you are able to straighten your legs, you can increase your range by gently holding on to your legs, wherever you can reach, and pulling them in the direction of your ears.

ENLIST YOUR MIND

Monitor your chin. Identify the shortening feeling in the back of your neck when the chin starts creeping up to the ceiling. Spare it half a thought—and then adjust it downward to relax the back of the neck. Develop this wider sense of body position. As you do, it will become second nature.

SAFETY NOTE

Make sure your body is adequately prepared to undertake this demanding stretch: perhaps even enlist an experienced instructor's guidance. Attempting this position too quickly can result in injury.

KEY

Erector spinae:
- Longissimus thoracis
- Iliocostalis

- Semitendinosus
- Biceps femoris (long head)
- Biceps femoris (short head)

back

61

PART TWO YOUR STRETCH REPERTORY

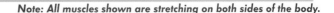

Note: All muscles shown are stretching on both sides of the body.

12 lower back (flexion): chest to thighs, kneeling

ENLIST YOUR MIND

Imagine that someone is ironing your back in long, gentle, warm strokes. Send your tailbone down toward your feet. Relax the upper part of your back. Allow your back to increase its length for as long as you hold the position.

- **The Setup:** This stretch is the flip side of stretch 11a, "Knees to Chest." It carries a bit more intensity than the first stretch, because your body weight is now pressing your chest closer to your thighs, which creates more length in your back than you can get by pulling your knees into your chest, as in stretch 11a.

  Start by kneeling on the floor and open your knees a bit. Flatten your feet (toes are not tucked on this one).

- **The Stretch:** Let your butt sink back toward your heels. See how far back you can take your butt. You have gained a good amount of flexibility when you feel your butt touching your heels.

  Choose your arm and head position: (1) reach your arms forward and place your forehead on the floor; (2) cross your elbows in front of you and rest your forehead on your forearms; or (3) position your arms at your sides and rest your forehead on the floor.

- **Enhance Your Flexibility:** See if you can locate your sacrum using your inside radar and gently flatten it, so that your abdomen and chest come closer to your thighs. This will increase the stretch and develop awareness of sacral movement. If you can sense your sacrum and lower back moving up and away from your hips and legs, your ability to flex your spine farther and farther forward will grow. This feeling is a tool you can use to overcome stiffness and create a fluid lower-back/hamstring connection.

KEY

Erector spinae:

- Iliocostalis
- Longissimus
- Spinalis thoracis

Multifidi

Note: All muscles shown are stretching on both sides of the body.

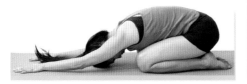

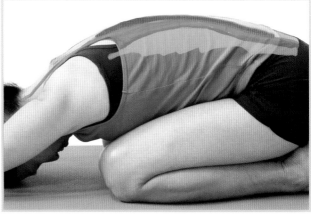

13 lower back (flexion): backward pull, seated

- **The Setup:** Here you are still targeting the same muscles you lengthened in stretches 11a–c and stretch 12. You may find one stretch more effective than another, because every body is different. In this lower-back/sacrum stretch group you have several choices to try out.

    This particular position uses your body's own leverage to create the stretchy feeling.

    Sit on the floor with both legs straight out in front of you. Flex both feet; bend your knees slightly; open your toes to the side. If you were to stand up, you would be using Charlie Chaplin's signature pose, or standing in the first position in ballet, with a little plié.

- **The Stretch:** Grab your heels with your hands. It's fine if you cannot reach your heels: just hold onto your legs as far down as you can without too much discomfort. Keeping a firm grip on your heels or legs, drop your head down between your arms and relax your neck. Your view is your belly button.

    Lean gently back, away from the pull of your hands. Look for the stretchy feeling, as before, in the area of your waistline and below. Slow pulsing or static holding work well with this stretch (see *Part One: Ways to Stretch*, p. 31).

- **Enhance Your Flexibility:** This stretch, more than the others in the section, has a specific focus at the waistline. When you first experience its power, you may realize that your back has been asleep in this spot. Wake it up with care. Judge how much pull to exert, as your body settles in and learns how to feel this stretch.

ENLIST YOUR MIND

Here is a legitimate chance to slump! You may have been told so many times to sit up straight in school that you no longer know how to do it. Here slumping is actually beneficial to your back's flexibility. For an effective stretch, lean backward and imagine that your waistline area is lit up with a calming color. (Try blue for relaxation and peace, or turquoise to calm and soothe.)

KEY

Erector spinae:

- Iliocostalis
- Longissimus
- Spinalis thoracis

- Multifidi

Note: All muscles shown are stretching on both sides of the body.

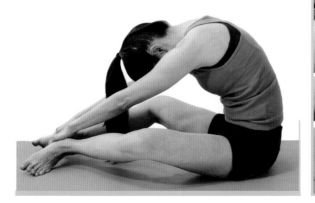

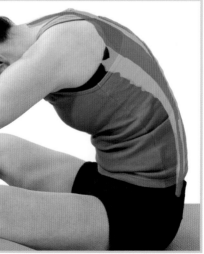

14 lower back (flexion): hug and release, seated

- **The Setup:** Sit on the floor with your knees bent and feet in front of you. Hug your elbows around your thighs; grab each opposite elbow with your hands. Pull your chest right to the thighs. Bend your knees as much as you need to in order to feel your chest actually touching your thighs. You may already be experiencing the lifting-up feeling in your lower-back/sacral area. Relax your head forward so you do not tax the neck muscles.

- **The Stretch:** Very slowly, begin to straighten your legs. As you do, concentrate on keeping your thighs against your chest. Take as much time as you want to in your progress towards straightening your legs.

    At some point—farther away from the floor if you need more flexibility work, closer if you are more flexible to begin with—your chest will come away from your thighs. This is okay. Continue your slow descent toward the floor. When your legs become so straight that you have to release your arms from behind your legs, gently place your arms by your sides without disturbing your position.

    Stay in your final position a bit longer, reaching for the feeling of new length in your lower back and sacrum. This stretch works well when you perform it twice.

- **Enhance Your Flexibility:** The special character of this stretch will allow you to explore the feeling of length in your lower back and sacrum. Many stretches exist for this general area, but to make them effective you must first discover how to feel length in the area. Take your time with the stretch and let your body figure out this new feeling. It is an important key to attaining a flexible back.

Note: See left for the muscles stretched and opposite for how to do the stretch.

KEY

Erector spinae:

- Iliocostalis
- Longissimus
- Spinalis thoracis

- Multifidi

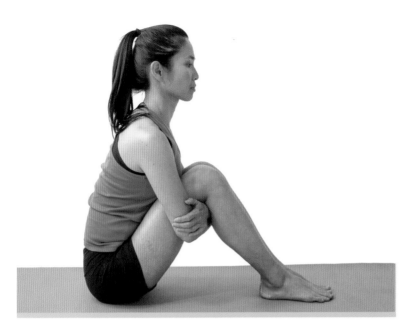

ENLIST YOUR MIND

Keep thinking: lift up, up and forward, up and forward. Be patient with your mind–body connection. If you discover that, when you gave the signal to lengthen your lower back, you have cricked your neck instead, then you know your body computer does not yet have a program for the thought you are sending it. Take a breath. Start again; repeat the signal. Leave it for the day; try it again the next day. You are educating your body to interpret the signals your mind sends it. You may be surprised at how much your body learned the next time you try this.

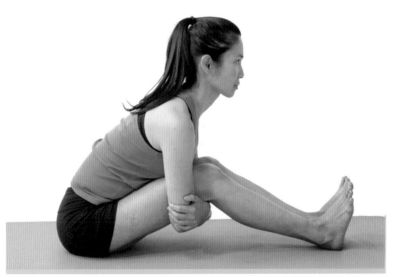

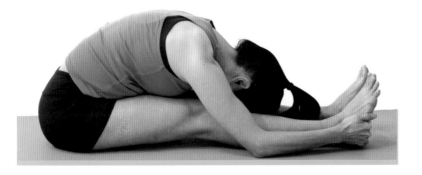

15 lower back (extension): chest and pelvic lift

ENLIST YOUR MIND

To develop a clear understanding of what you are lengthening, here's what to think:

- Lift sacrum to the ceiling to create the low-back extension.
- Lift chest to the ceiling to create the upper-back extension.
- Gently press knees together to create stretch across the low spine.
- Lift sacrum to its highest point to feel hip-flexor length.

KEY

Erector spinae:

▣ Iliocostalis

▣ Longissimus

Multifidi

▣ Tensor fascia lata

▣ Sartorius

Note: In the illustration shown here, some of the back muscles being stretched overlay the arm. All muscles shown are stretching on both sides of the body.

- **The Setup:** Lie on your back on the floor, using a carpet or a mat for comfort. Bend your knees and place both feet on the floor. Place your arms by your sides, palms down. Open your feet wider than your knees, and test the range by pressing your knees inwards. If your knees touch, open your feet a bit wider. When you go into the stretch and bring your knees together, you want to be able to get to the end of your knees' range without having them contact each other.

- **The Stretch:** Lift your chest up onto your shoulders. You may have to adjust your shoulders a bit forward or toward each other, to make sure your chest is well supported. Make sure your neck remains relaxed. You should be resting your lifted chest on your shoulders. Then, lift your sacrum and low spine up into the air. Lift as high as you can; then bring your knees together at the height of the stretch.

  In this stretch, you are creating a beautiful spinal-extension arc in your back. Reach for the feeling of stretch all along your back— from upper back to sacrum. Bringing your knees together will also create a widening stretch across your sacrum and lower back. Last, as you lift your sacrum toward the ceiling, look for stretch in your hip-flexor area—just where your hips crease in front.

- **Enhance Your Flexibility:** Keep any strain away from your low back by concentrating on lifting the chest and the sacrum at the same time. Experiment with the different parts of this stretch gently. There are several different stretches happening here. This may be new territory for you, so you may feel sore in unaccustomed places the day after trying this technique.

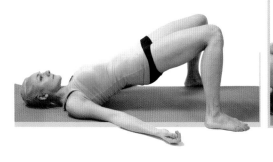

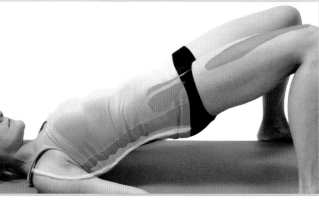

16 lower back (extension): sacrum lift, kneeling

back

ENLIST YOUR MIND

Always think "up and forward," not just "forward." This will keep your back lengthening through its many vertebrae. You will never be in danger of compressing the vertebrae together.

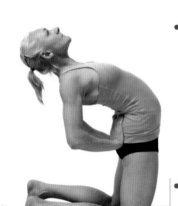

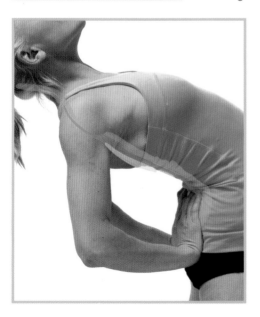

- **The Setup:** Kneel on the floor, using a carpet or mat if needed. When you execute any stretch, your body should feel comfortable. Tuck your toes. Place your hands behind you at sacrum/lower-back level.

  Here's the tricky part. Your palms should be facing your body, with the fingertips lifting the sacrum up and out of the pelvis. You might get into this position (which does feel strange at first) by starting with your hands by your sides with the palms facing back. Lift your fingers up so that your wrists extend, and move your hands behind your back, allowing your fingers to touch your spine. They should land in the area of the sacrum/lower back.

- **The Stretch:** Allow your fingers to give you the feeling of sacrum/lower-back lift, as you send them gently upward. Let your shoulders drop down and back and your chest lift as you feel your back lengthen into extension. Your neck follows the curve of the rest of your back. This stretch lends itself particularly to the breathing rhythm of exhale/lift the fingers, inhale/relax the finger lift. You can also press upward and hold in a gentle static stretch. Expect to feel some stretch in the hip-flexor area as well, where your hips crease in front.

- **Enhance Your Flexibility:** Become aware of the degree of curve made by your entire spine. Your neck (cervical spine) is part of that curve. It should curve only as much as the rest of your spine is capable of doing, and no more. Most people's neck curves have greater range than their back curves. A common mistake is thinking that you are curving your spine more by cricking your neck. This will just strain your neck, potentially causing problems with it. Instead, work on developing an accurate sense of the curve of your whole back. From this initial awareness you can progress to greater back extension range.

KEY

▤ Semispinalis capitis

Erector spinae:

▤ Iliocostalis

▤ Longissimus

▢ Spinalis thoracis

Note: On the artwork shown here, some of the back muscles being stretched overlay the shoulder and hand. All muscles shown are stretching on both sides of the body.

17 lower back (extension): towel under pelvis

- **The Setup:** Lie comfortably on your back, with a carpet or a mat to cushion you, if you like. (To discourage ribcage arch, rest your arms by your sides.) Place a rolled-up towel under the curve of your lower back, just opposite your belly button.

- **The Stretch:** This is a stretch in which you can just relax and let gravity do the work. Once the towel is in place, allow your pelvis to relax into the floor below the towel, and your ribs to relax into the floor above the towel. Breathe deeply and regularly as you relax around your new lower-back curve. That's it. Just breathe and enjoy.

- **Enhance Your Flexibility:** The bigger the towel, the more your lower back will lift. If you have never experienced lower-back extension, this may be an unfamiliar feeling. In my own case, I was made so afraid of crunching my vertebrae together that I left lower-back extension out of my stretching repertory for a long time. Slowly get used to feeling a greater lower-back curve, and progress to a thicker towel roll as you learn to relax and let the curve happen.

ENLIST YOUR MIND

Here you have a chance to develop awareness both of your pelvis and your ribcage. If you have any sense of your ribs sticking up into the air, just keep talking to them and feel them against the floor when they let go. Your thought is: ribs and pelvis sink and relax.

KEY

Erector spinae:

Iliocostalis

Longissimus cervicis, thoracis

Spinalis thoracis

Rectus abdominis
External oblique

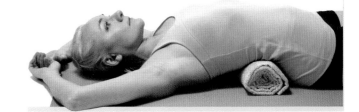

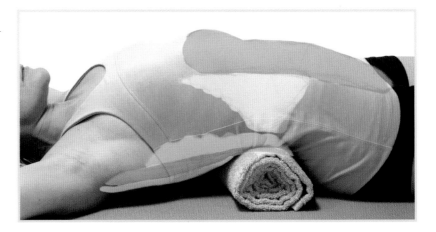

Note: All muscles shown are stretching on both sides of the body.

18 upper back (flexion): crossed-elbows hug

ENLIST YOUR MIND

ENLIST YOUR MIND

Spare half a thought for your knees. Check that they have not crept up into the locked-out position. Keep them relaxed and slightly bent throughout.

- **The Setup:** Stand with your feet comfortably apart, about the width of your shoulders. Keep your knees slightly bent throughout the stretch. As you move into the stretch position, let your neck relax and your gaze drop.

- **The Stretch:** Cross your elbows at shoulder height. Reach your fingers as far around your shoulders as you can. If you can actually grab onto the inside edges of your shoulder blades, you will have a solid place to anchor your fingers.

  Slowly round your upper back and let it expand backward between your fingers. This is called "hollow back." To execute this position, you need a degree of body awareness. You must teach your body, in effect, how to do this hollowing. It is okay if you also feel your lower back rounding in response to the action of your upper back. You are just not concentrating the stretch there. Your pelvis can remain in neutral (neither tucked nor tilted) or slightly tucked. Just keep feeling for the stretch in your upper back.

- **Enhance Your Flexibility:** As your upper back widens in this stretch, you may be able to feel your shoulder blades actually separating a little, sliding outward along your ribcage. You can encourage this action with your fingers. You are not trying to pull the bones off your body—just to create a little more width in your back.

KEY
- Rhomboids
- Trapezius
- Latissimus dorsi

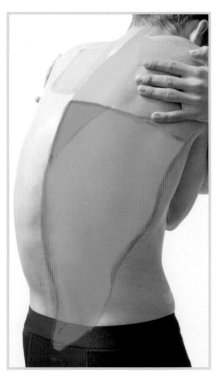

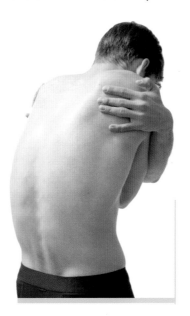

Note: In the illustration shown here, some of the back muscles being stretched overlay the hand. All muscles shown are stretching on both sides of the body.

19 upper back (flexion): backward pull, standing

ENLIST YOUR MIND

Begin thinking about being able to tuck and tilt your pelvis. When you can do that, the next thing is being able to tuck and tilt your pelvis while keeping your ribs stationary. (See p. 58 for an introduction to these concepts.) Of course these are movements for your body to do, but the first step in your ability to do a movement is a clear understanding of what that movement is.

KEY

Rhomboids
Trapezius
Latissimus dorsi

- **The Setup:** Stand with your feet comfortably apart, about the width of your shoulders. Keep your knees slightly bent throughout the stretch. As you move into the stretch position, let your neck relax and your gaze drop.

  For this stretch, you will be leaning backward against a support that doesn't move. Some possibilities in your home may be (a) a doorway with mouldings on either side that extend out from the wall and form convenient finger holds; (b) a floor-to-ceiling stationary pole; or (c) two doorknobs on either side of an open door. Even a stretching partner holding the other end of a towel, as shown here, can work, if the person leans back and counters your pull.

- **The Stretch:** Grasp your support firmly at approximately shoulder height, and slowly lean away from it, rounding your upper back and letting it expand backward. You are creating a "hollow back." To get in touch with the widening feeling of this stretch, just keep imagining that you can feel your upper back getting broader. You may need to try the position several times, perhaps on different days, to allow your body time to learn how to execute it well.

  This stretch is a more intense version of stretch 18, so you may want to try that one first. As in that stretch, don't be too concerned if you feel your lower back responding to your commands for your upper back. Just keep concentrating on what's happening in your upper back.

- **Enhance Your Flexibility:** Experiment with adjusting (a) your pelvis forward or backward a little; (b) your feet the same; and (c) the height of your hands a little higher or lower. Concentrate on the stretchy feeling in your upper back, and how it is increased or diminished as you make these little adjustments. Discover the optimal stretch position for your body.

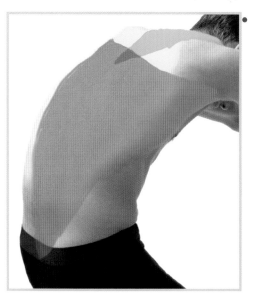

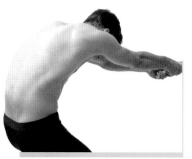

Note: All muscles shown are stretching on both sides of the body.

20 upper back (extension): towel under ribs

- **The Setup:** Lie comfortably on your back, with a carpet or a mat to cushion you, if you like. Your arms are resting by your sides. Place a rolled-up towel under your upper back, just at your chest line. For women, this will be your bra line; for men, the line of your nipples.

- **The Stretch:** This is another stretch using gravity to create upper-back extension length. All that is required is that you allow your ribs to relax below the spot where the towel rests. Slow, steady, deep breathing is your friend here. Increase to a thicker towel when your body adapts to the one you began with.

- **Enhance Your Flexibility:** The human back wants to expand— in every direction—simply because increased range feels good. As you practice this stretch and allow your back to get used to lengthening in extension, your back may thank you by letting you experience increased extension range. This is the opposite of a vicious cycle. You ask your body for length. It realizes you have its best interests in mind and complies with more length. And the next round—more flexibility.

ENLIST YOUR MIND

Imagine your ribs and the tops of your shoulders melting, and sinking down to the floor on the upper and lower sides of the towel. Feel the small curve in your lower back, and send a quiet command to your pelvis to relax as well.

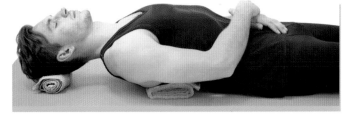

Note: In the illustration shown here, some of the back muscles being stretched overlay the arm. All muscles shown are stretching on both sides of the body.

KEY

Erector spinae:

- Iliocostalis
- Longissimus

- Multifidi
- Rectus abdominis
- External oblique

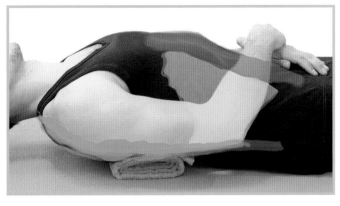

21 upper back (extension): arms long, all fours

- **The Setup:** Get into the all-fours position on the floor. Your body is a table top: knees under butt, hands under shoulders.

- **The Stretch:** Keeping your butt over your knees, extend your arms forward. Sink your chest through your shoulders to create extension in your upper back. As you create more stretch in this area, you will be able to extend your arms farther forward, causing your butt to come forward of your knees. Check on your neck, making sure you are not thrusting your chin forward and causing a crick in your neck. Gaze downward, or along the line of the floor, to let your neck relax.

  You are working on developing the feeling of gently sinking your chest through your shoulders. If all you feel is shoulder stretch, and no upper-back stretch, come back to this stretch when you have created more length in the front of your shoulders (stretches 6–9).

- **Enhance Your Flexibility:** The feeling of sinking your chest through your shoulders is an unfamiliar one for many people. The upper-back area is addressed less often in stretch routines. Since lower-back problems commonly abound, the average person will normally encounter those stretches more often. You may experience some soreness in this area when you first work on opening up your upper back. As long as you work gently, this should pass.

ENLIST YOUR MIND

This is a more intense version of stretch 20. It is a good idea to practice stretch 20 before proceeding to this stretch. Then carry the feeling of your upper back curving over the towel in your mind, and remind your body of that feeling when you practice this one.

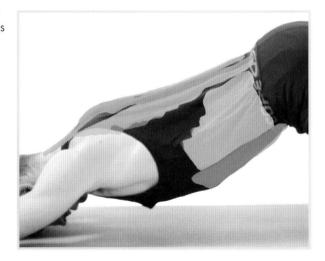

KEY

Erector spinae:

Iliocostalis

Longissimus

Multifidi

External oblique

Rectus abdominis

Note: All muscles shown are stretching on both sides of the body.

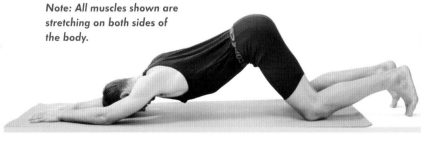

22 full spine: extension (sphinx)

ENLIST YOUR MIND

Increase the effect of this stretch by picturing your spinal column and its vertebral discs. They are separated by a cushion of cerebrospinal fluid, which lubricates the joints and creates ease and fluidity in your movement. As you execute gentle self-traction, imagine those discs pulling slightly more apart, allowing more fluid in to cushion movement.

KEY

Erector spinae:

- Iliocostalis
- Longissimus

- Multifidi
- External oblique
- Rectus abdominis

Note: In the illustration shown here, some of the muscles being stretched overlay the arm. All muscles shown are stretching on both sides of the body.

- **The Setup:** Lie on your stomach on the floor, using a mat or carpet for comfort. Begin with your arms extended in front of you, palms down. Lift your head slightly off the floor, with your neck long: you are gazing down at the floor. Your legs are long, with your feet stretching out behind you.

- **The Stretch:** Take a breath, and as you do, let your chest lift a little from the floor, making a slight upward curve with your neck and head. As you exhale, begin to move through an upper-body wave with the top of your head leading. Your head dips forward and comes up, followed slowly by your chin, your neck, your chest, your shoulders. As you create this wave, and your chest begins to lift off the floor, draw your straight arms back along the floor, creating a pull as your forearms head for their destination directly under your shoulders. Throughout the stretch duration, this gentle pull backward of the forearms continues.

  Once your forearms are in place under your shoulders, keep them there. The pull backward is isometric: your arms are not actually going to move, just exert pressure backward so your upper-back muscles will contract, creating traction and length all the way down your back. Enhance this feeling of back length by stretching your toes out behind you.

  Roll your shoulders down to lift your chest, and lift the back of your neck to create length. Slowly turn your head to the left. Feel how this adds extra length to your spine. Slowly return your head to the center. Repeat the head turn to the right.

- **Enhance Your Flexibility:** The main purpose of this stretch is to create extra space between the vertebrae of your spine. This will give you ease and freedom when you move, and make injury from sudden movements less likely. As you hold the stretch, continuing to create gentle spinal self-traction, look for an elusive sense of "well-being" when your sacral and lower-back vertebrae decompress. You may feel "relief" or "release"—or just surprise when you stand up and feel taller.

back

73

PART TWO YOUR STRETCH REPERTORY

23 full spine: side, using chair

KEY

Erector spinae:

▢ Iliocostalis

▣ Longissimus

▢ Multifidi
   External oblique

- **The Setup:** Sit on a stool or in a chair with your knees bent and feet on a stool rung or on the floor. Keep your shoulders facing forward; be sure you don't turn them to the side. Lift your left arm up at your side, palm facing inward. Grasp a stool or chair leg with your right hand. Look straight ahead. It may be helpful to check your position in a mirror.

- **The Stretch:** Begin to reach your long left arm slowly to the right. Counter the weight shift created by pressing your left sitting bone down onto the stool or chair. You will feel the stretch in your left side. As you lean farther to the right, you will be able to move your right hand farther down the stool or chair leg and feel more stretch. Try pulling upward with your right hand to see if that will increase your feeling of stretch. Your neck curve matches the curve of your arm. Repeat on the other side.

  Your goal here is to feel the stretch along the left side of your torso. If you feel it in your arm instead, try settling your shoulder into its socket to relax your arm. It takes a little practice to master the feeling of a long arm that is reaching but not working. Instead the back supports it—in this case the side of the back.

- **Enhance Your Flexibility:** To get the right placement of your head relative to your arm, bring up your right arm to complete the oval shape begun by the left arm, and place your head exactly in the center of the two. When you return your right arm to its position on the stool or chair rung, your head should exactly match the curve of your left arm.

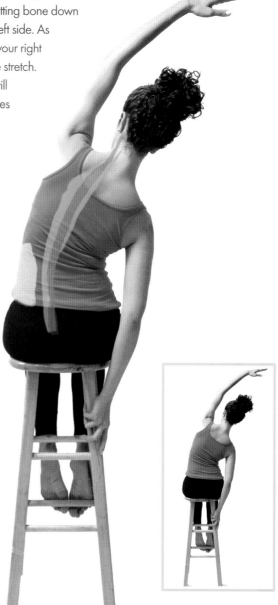

ENLIST YOUR MIND

Remember that any stretch is created by pulling two points on the body apart, and lengthening the muscles between those points. Here the two points to imagine pulling away from each other are your left fingertips and your left sitting bone.

24a spiral: both knees to side, supine

Along with stretches 22 and 23, this group of three stretches addresses the full length of your spine. You may find 24a the gentlest. To add a little more intensity, experiment with 24b. The 24c position is not necessarily more intense or more advanced; rather, because you're sitting up and using your arms to help your body stretch, it requires more effort and is less relaxing.

- **The Setup:** Lie on your back on the floor, using a carpet or mat for comfort. Place your arms by your side, palms down, forming an "A" shape (fingers reaching away from you at 45 degrees to your torso).

- **The Stretch:** Bring both your knees as far in to your chest as you can. Drop both knees over to the left side and let them rest where they fall. Keep your right shoulder down on the floor. The stretch here is produced by your knees pulling away from your shoulder, causing your spine to form its characteristic spiral shape. Repeat the stretch on the other side.

- **Enhance Your Flexibility:** This is the first stretch in this spiral series in terms of intensity. If your right knee is resting directly on top of your left knee, you have reached the maximum spiral stretch in this position. To add more intensity to your spiral, go on to stretches 24b and 24c.

  If your right knee is hanging above the left one but not reaching it yet, it is okay. Any stretch requires practice, and learning things would be no fun if everything worked perfectly immediately. There will likely be a strong pull across your lower spine. If you can hold this pull without grimacing, allow the weight of your leg to bring your knee down gradually until, with enough familiarity with this stretch, your body is able to rest the right knee on top of the left. If the pull feels too strong at the moment, just place your left hand under your right knee. Give the knee as much support as it needs, so that you still feel a strong pull across your back, but not so much that you can think of nothing else.

ENLIST YOUR MIND

There will be some stretches you can do easily, and some that will challenge you and show you where your overall flexibility needs more work. This is true even for the most accomplished and advanced flexibility practitioner. Stretching is a life-long journey. Try on the thought that you may come to love those stretches most that contributed most to your learning experience—the ones that initially cost you a struggle.

Note: All back muscles shown are stretching on both sides of the body.

KEY

- Gluteus maximus
- External oblique
- Iliocostalis
- Gluteus medius
- Longissimus

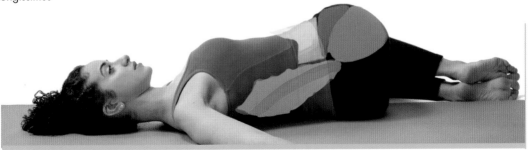

24b spiral: knee crossed over body, supine

- **The Setup:** Lie on your back on the floor, using a carpet or mat for comfort. Place your arms by your sides, palms down, forming an "A" shape (fingers reaching away from you at 45 degrees to your torso).

ENLIST YOUR MIND

In flexibility training, you will always be dealing with degrees of intensity in the stretchy feeling. That feeling will always be with you, even when you have a perfect 180-degree side split. It is the characteristic feeling you get when muscles stretch. When you are deciding how intense to let the stretchy feeling become, consider your body's comfort.

You and your body are in partnership in your flexibility training adventure. Bodies are very smart, and they don't like feeling pain. A body will always move away from pain—it's hard-wired that way to survive. Your body will be more likely to join your mind in achieving a common flexibility goal if you succeed in making stretching enjoyable for it. Just like your mind, if stretching is something your body likes and looks forward to doing, it is more likely to seek that experience, simply because it feels good. Of course, there is some crash-course training that takes stretching into the realm of pain, but I believe there are better ways to become flexible.

- **The Stretch:** Bring your right knee in to your chest as far as you can. Keep your left leg straight and in line with your hips: be careful that the left leg does not creep out more to the left. Cross your right knee over your body and let it fall to the left. You will feel the stretch diagonally across your back, especially in your lower spine. Make sure your foot is not resting on your leg. Repeat the stretch on the other side.

- **Enhance Your Flexibility:** Your right knee may touch the floor, or it may be suspended above it. Again, as in stretch 24a, use your left hand to give the right knee the support it needs, depending on the intensity of the pull across your back.

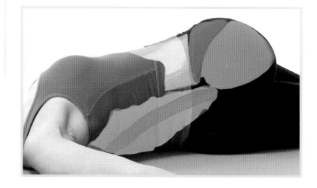

KEY

- Gluteus maximus
- External oblique
- Iliocostalis
- Gluteus medius
- Longissimus

Note: Back muscles shown are stretching on both sides of the body.

24c spiral: seated, using special arm positions

ENLIST YOUR MIND

Here you are always thinking: back lifts up and around; chest lifts up; shoulders drop. A good image for your brain is the barbershop pole, whose stripes spiral endlessly upward. That's what your spine does in this position. Keep thinking how it turns, how all the little muscles close to the spine enable it to spiral continuously up and up, as long as you hold the stretch. Your spine is a marvelous thing.

- **The Setup:** Sit on the floor, on a carpet or mat for comfort if you like. Stretch both legs out in front of you. Flex both feet; bend the right knee slightly, so that your right heel is about 6 in (15 cm) behind your left heel.

- **The Stretch:** Reach your left arm across your right knee. It will come to rest against your knee somewhere below your elbow. Your left arm will create one-half of the stretch. Place your right arm behind your back, right next to your spine. Rotate your fingers outward (backward) so that your shoulder follows and rotates down and backward. This action allows your chest to lift as your shoulder drops. Your right arm will create the other half of the stretch. Finally, look over your right shoulder.

    Press your right knee with your left arm, and press your right hand to the floor. Your shoulders will turn; your chest will lift as you drop the right shoulder; and you will look like the figures in an Egyptian painting—torso facing front, head in profile. Look for the stretchy feeling anywhere from lowest to highest point in your spine. It will show up in the spots where your spine needs most flexibility. Repeat the stretch on the other side.

- **Enhance Your Flexibility:** Crucial to the success of this stretch is the position of your right arm: right up against your back. This prevents any possibility of your leaning back. You are embracing your spine between your two arms and using your own body as the leverage to create the stretch. It may seem paradoxical as you sit in this upright position, but your spine can actually learn to relax and rest even when it lifts, as your two arms twine around it.

Note: See stretch 24b, opposite, for illlustration of muscles stretching.

Abdominals

In this section we will cover stretches for the major abdominal muscles—which pull the spine into flexion, rotate the torso, and support it. The two stretches described here address all the relevant abdominal muscles. Abdominals also stretch in: lower-back extension—stretches 15–17; upper-back extension—stretches 20–21; and full spine—stretches 22–24.

Causes of stiff, sore, or aching abdominal muscles/muscles in spasm	• Using your abdominal muscles to support your torso in an awkward position—such as reaching underneath a sink or bathtub to clean the area. This is a case of sustained muscular effort: you must hold yourself in the position long enough to get the area clean.
	• Strenuous or unaccustomed physical activity—such as your first attempts at doing pull-ups. Although pull-ups primarily involve back strength, the abdominals are heavily engaged, and the resulting post-exercise soreness may take you by surprise.
	• Playing sports or doing activities that require a lot of core engagement—basketball, golf, running, walking, chopping wood.
	• Playing sports or doing activities that require a lot of torso rotation—golf, racquetball/handball, throwing sports, chopping wood.
Injuries eased by stretching	• Abdominal muscle strain.
	• Hip-flexor strain.
	• Iliopsoas (hip-flexor) tendonitis.
Additional uses	• Before and after playing sports requiring extensive core engagement or torso rotation—basketball, golf, racquetball/handball, running, throwing sports, walking.
	• To relieve stiff back muscles: doing abdominal stretches may also help with back soreness.

Pinpoint the area of discomfort (this connects your mind with your body), and choose the stretch that most closely reaches that spot.

For guidance on stretch duration, see pp. 32–33. To discover how to use breathing to deepen the stretch, see pp. 34–35.

25 abdominals: finger-and-toe reach, supine

- **The Setup:** Lie on your back on a comfortable floor, complete with carpet or mat if you like. Stretch your legs out long, and your arms overhead, letting them extend along the floor behind your head.

- **The Stretch:** Point your toes and reach them away from your torso as far as you can. Feel your legs get longer. Reach your fingers along the floor behind you, allowing your arms to get longer as well. You will feel the stretch in the abdominal space between legs and arms. The space will elongate and hollow out.

  This stretch lends itself to a slow, inhale/exhale breathing rhythm. Inhale: gather yourself for the stretch. Exhale: reach your upper and lower limbs away from each other. Make each breath a long, deliberate one.

- **Enhance Your Flexibility:** Experiment with variations on this stretch. Stretch your right hand and right leg away from each other, while the left side relaxes. Feel how much longer your right side becomes. Then do the same on the left side. Also try reaching the right hand and left leg away from each other, to create a diagonal stretch feeling across your abdominal area.

ENLIST YOUR MIND

Imagine that your toes are starting a chain reaction of length in your legs, and that your pelvis follows the legs away from your torso, creating extra space in your abdominal cavity. Likewise, think of your fingers starting the same chain reaction of length all along your arms down to your shoulders. Allow your shoulders to lift away from your ribs, creating abdominal space from above.

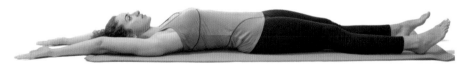

KEY

▢ External oblique
▢ Rectus abdominis
▢ Transversus abdominis

Note: All muscles shown are stretching on both sides of the body.

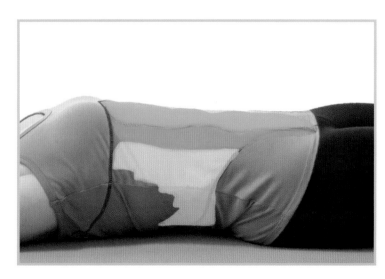

26 abdominals: torso lift from floor, using arms

- **The Setup:** Lie on the floor on your stomach. Place your hands, palms down, under your shoulders.

- **The Stretch:** Slowly push your hands against the floor, gradually straightening your arms. This stretch also requires an ability to extend the low spine. If you feel mostly low spine and not abdominals stretching, practice stretches 15–17 and 22 first. Then come back to this one and see if you can locate the abdominal stretch feeling.

- **Enhance Your Flexibility:** You may need several repetitions of this stretch during a session before you can straighten your arms all the way. This is okay. Take as much time as you need to reach the full stretch. You may also build up to full range over several days or a week of practice.

ENLIST YOUR MIND

Develop your thought path: shoulders rolling down and relaxing back. Pubic bone sinking toward the floor. Those two points—shoulders and pubic bone—drawing away from each other create length up the front of your torso. Neck rises long out of the shoulders as they sink.

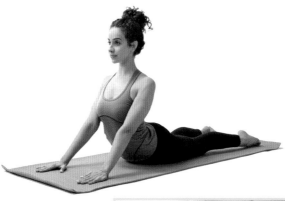

KEY
- Rectus abdominis
- Transversus abdominis
- External oblique

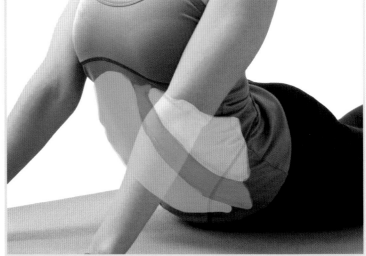

Note: In the illustration shown here, some of the abdominal muscles being stretched overlay the arm. All muscles shown are stretching on both sides of the body.

Arms, wrists, and hands

In this section we will cover stretches for the biceps (front of the arm), triceps (back of the arm), wrists (affecting forearms), and hands. You may be surprised how much better your hands and wrists feel with just a few minutes of daily stretching.

Causes of stiff, sore, or aching arm and hand muscles/muscles in spasm	• Holding your hand in a fixed position—such as: —Grasping your phone throughout a long conversation. —Holding the computer mouse for long periods. —Clenching your paintbrush, pencil, or crayon too tightly while mastering drawing or painting techniques. —Holding onto a pole on public transport, or gripping the steering wheel of your car during a stressful commute. —Carrying weight in your arms—for example, a child. • Repetitive motions (that may also require strength) in an occupation—such as: —Performing massage therapy. —Practicing a musical instrument. Violin playing is a classic case. The left hand and arm are fixed in an awkward position, while the fingers must be dexterous. The right hand maintains a fixed position on the bow. (Actually, this is an example of repetitive motion for the left hand and a fixed position for the right.)
Injuries eased by stretching	• Bicepital tendonitis. • Biceps strain. • Elbow strain or mild sprain. • Golfer's elbow. • Tennis elbow. • Thrower's elbow. • Wrist sprain (mild). • Wrist tendonitis. • Carpal tunnel syndrome.
Additional uses	• Before and after playing sports requiring either a fixed hold on a piece of equipment (like racquetball) or constant/intense use of the hands (like basketball)—i.e., racquet or ball-handling sports. • Before and after playing sports or doing activities requiring extensive full-arm use—such as swimming and throwing sports. • To prevent pain in elbow and wrist joints, since the arm and forearm muscles are used so frequently.

Pinpoint the area of discomfort (this connects your mind with your body), and choose the stretch that most closely reaches that spot.

For guidance on stretch duration, see pp. 32–33. To discover how to use breathing to deepen the stretch, see pp. 34–35.

27 triceps: elbow behind head

ENLIST YOUR MIND

Monitor your ribcage—make sure you are not thrusting it forward. Keep it in line with the rest of your torso. If you're standing, make sure your knees maintain a gentle bend and don't lock out.

- **The Setup:** Sit or stand comfortably. If you're sitting, place both feet on the floor next to each other; if standing, place your feet shoulder width apart with knees slightly bent. Raise your left arm straight up at your side, with your palm facing front.

- **The Stretch:** Reach up with your right hand and grasp your left elbow. Gently pull your left elbow downward. The stretch will appear in the back of your left arm, between your elbow and your shoulder (triceps area). Repeat the stretch on the other side.

- **Enhance Your Flexibility:** The area of stretch will probably be immediately evident. This is a good stretch for a steady, continuous pull. Your elbow will gradually move farther down as you hold the stretch.

  Be aware of your head and whether it has to bow forward to accommodate your arm behind it. Try to straighten your head against your arm, and notice if you encounter resistance in the front of your left shoulder. If you find it challenging to straighten your head, stop and stretch the front of your shoulder first (stretches 6 and 7). When you return to this stretch, you will have more freedom of range in your shoulder, which will allow your arm to move farther back and your head to come up more easily.

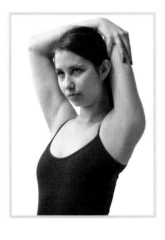

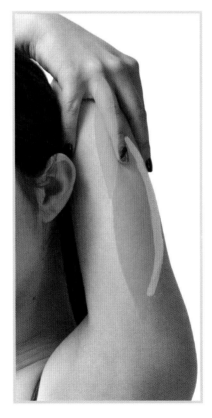

Note: In the illustration shown here, some of the arm muscles being stretched overlay the fingers.

KEY

▪ Triceps (long head)
▪ Triceps (lateral head)
▪ Triceps (medial head)

28 triceps: finger or towel pull

- **The Setup:** Sit or stand comfortably as in stretch 27. Your feet are either side by side on the floor if you're sitting, or shoulder width apart if you're standing. Raise your right arm straight up at your side, with your palm facing front. Bend your elbow: your right hand will reach down your back.

- **The Stretch: Finger Pull.** Bend your left elbow, and place the back of your left hand against your back. Reach your right hand down toward your left, and your left hand up toward your right. The stretch is complete when the fingers of each hand are pulling securely against each other—right fingers pull up against the left; left fingers pull down against the right. The feeling of stretch will be in the back of your right arm (as in stretch 27). Repeat the stretch on the other side.

- **The Stretch: Towel Pull.** Your preparation is the same as for the "Finger Pull." For the greater stretch it requires, you can use a towel to develop sufficient flexibility in your triceps (of both arms). A hand towel is a good size. Grasp one end of the rolled-up towel with each hand and pause to feel the stretch in your triceps. Repeat the stretch on the other side.

- **Enhance Your Flexibility:** Here you are challenging not only the right arm to stretch the triceps, but also the left arm, which must also be flexible enough in the triceps and shoulder. If you are teaching your body to stretch using a towel, you will gradually be able to move your hands closer together—one hand inching up and the other down the towel.

ENLIST YOUR MIND

Notice where your areas of stiffness lie. Here you have a chance to compare the flexibility of your right and left sides, because both are stretching simultaneously. In order to improve this stretch and make both sides more evenly flexible, you may need to give one side or the other a little extra flexibility attention. Any insight you gain into your body's current state will improve your partnership with your amazing body as you create easy, fluid movement.

KEY

- Triceps (lateral head)
- Triceps (long head)
- Triceps (medial head)

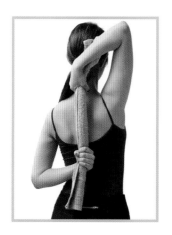
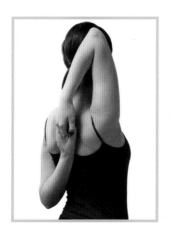
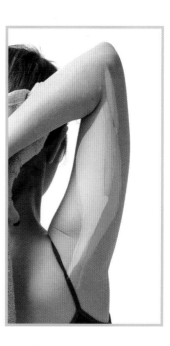

29 biceps: rotation, using pole

- **The Setup:** Stand sideways next to a pole or other upright support—preferably something around which you can securely wrap your fingers. (In a pinch, the side of an open door will do.) Extend your left arm straight out sideways. Turn your thumb down so your palm is facing back, and grasp your support with your fingers. As always, make sure your neck is relaxed, and your feet shoulder width apart with your knees slightly bent.

- **The Stretch:** Keeping your arm straight, try to rotate your upper arm (biceps) upward to face the ceiling. You will not get much of a movement—but you will get a good feeling of stretch. Repeat the stretch on the other side.

- **Enhance Your Flexibility:** This is a challenging stretch to feel, probably because stretching the biceps is not a common thing for most people. Knowing a biceps stretch is useful for a well-rounded stretching program. If the feeling of stretch eludes you here, try rotating your shoulder down and back, at the same time as you rotate your biceps upward. You can also try—carefully—a little stronger arm turn.

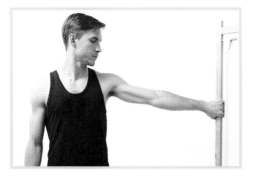

ENLIST YOUR MIND

Close your eyes as you make several efforts to rotate your arm and feel the stretch. You can also try reversing the position: turn your thumb up with your palm facing forward, and try to rotate your biceps downward, searching for the stretch with your mind.

KEY

- Biceps brachii
- Brachialis
- Pronator teres
- Brachioradialis

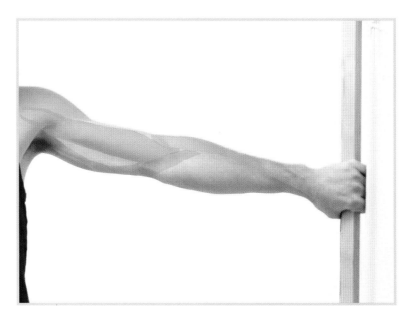

30 biceps: arm extended along wall

ENLIST YOUR MIND

Since your biceps area is an unfamiliar place to look for stretch, you may have to do some mental locating of the stretchy feeling. Be with the stretch for a while, seeking the feeling of stretch. Perhaps try it with the other arm. Often one side of our body can feel a stretch better, and then the other side will learn how to feel it from the side that already can.

- **The Setup:** Stand in a doorway, with a clear space of wall on each side wide enough to accommodate the whole length of your arm. Extend your left arm along this wall at shoulder height. Keep your arm straight and your palm flat on the wall. Place your shoulder at the edge of the doorway.

- **The Stretch:** Slowly turn your body away from your arm. Look for the stretch in the front of your upper arm—your biceps. Make sure your torso is aligned solidly over your legs, and that you are not sticking out your ribcage or tucking your pelvis under. Maintain a relaxed, shoulder-width stance of the feet as you gently create this biceps stretch. Repeat the stretch on the other side.

- **Enhance Your Flexibility:** Once you begin to feel the stretch in the correct spot, work on turning your body farther away from your outstretched arm—which is resting on the wall. Without forcing your body into any position, continue working on turning away from your arm, so that eventually you will be standing sideways in the doorway.

85

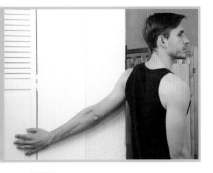

KEY

- Biceps brachii
- Brachialis
- Brachioradialis

Note: The muscles illustrated are on the inner arm but, for the purposes of illustration, are shown on the back of the arm.

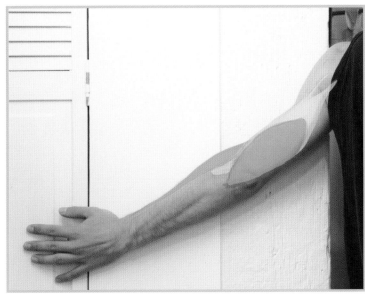

31 wrists: extension, fingers toward body

ENLIST YOUR MIND

Send a mental command to your inside elbows to keep them from hyper-extending. It is easy to feel that you are increasing the stretch in your wrists when you are just pushing your elbows forward. Check on your elbows from time to time as you hold the stretch. Your elbow position will soon become automatic.

Note: Double-jointed people should be especially careful with this stretch.

- **The Setup:** Kneel on the floor on all fours. Make your torso into a table top: hips over knees, shoulders over hands. Placing your palms down, turn your fingers toward your body in a straight line—not slanted.

- **The Stretch:** For many of us, the setup position is already quite a stretch. This isn't a position we normally find ourselves in. Lengthening the muscles in this area is beneficial as the years pass, if we want to keep the flexibility we were born with.

  Hold this position for your chosen stretch duration, breathing slowly and gently. You will feel the stretching sensation begin at your wrists and extend up into the front of your forearms.

- **Enhance Your Flexibility:** When you are ready for a bit more stretch, either move your hips backward, a little behind your knees, or move your arms forward, a little in front of your shoulders. Do whichever of these feels more comfortable. Extend your range a little at a time.

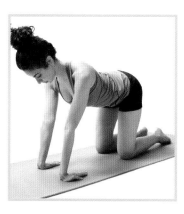

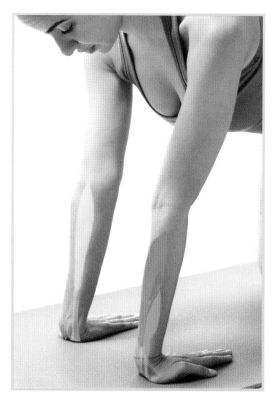

KEY

- Flexor pollicis longus
  Flexor digitorum profundus
- Flexor digitorum superficialis

Note: All muscles shown are stretching on both sides of the body.

32 wrists: flexion, fingers toward body

- **The Setup:** Kneel on the floor on all fours. Make your torso into a table top: hips over knees, shoulders over hands. Placing the backs of your hands down, turn your fingers toward your body in a straight line—not slanted.

- **The Stretch:** Hold this position for your chosen stretch duration, breathing slowly and gently. You will feel the stretching sensation begin at your wrists and extend up into the back of your forearms.

- **Enhance Your Flexibility:** As in stretch 31, when you are ready for a bit more stretch, either move your hips backward, a little behind your knees, or move your arms forward, a little in front of your shoulders, whichever feels more comfortable. Extend your range a little at a time.

ENLIST YOUR MIND

Although stretch 31 may initially be more challenging, we don't get into this position in our daily lives either. Take some calming breaths as you allow your mind to lessen its "running-away" feeling when it realizes the position you're asking the wrists to take. Imagine all the little muscle fibers in the back of your wrists lengthening and releasing tension.

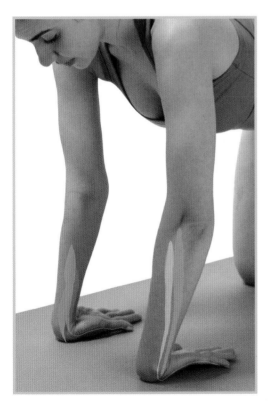

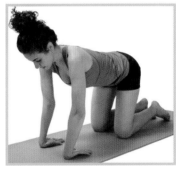

KEY

- ▨ Extensor carpi ulnaris
- ▨ Extensor pollicis brevis
- ▨ Extensor pollicis longus
- ▨ Extensor indicis
- ▨ Extensor digitorum

Note: All muscles shown are stretching on both sides of the body.

33 hands: finger extension

ENLIST YOUR MIND

If this stretch seems unfamiliar, it may help to close your eyes as you make adjustments and feel the stretch with your mind. Once you connect your mind to the stretch your body is feeling, the neural pathway is created, and the next time it will be much easier to locate the stretch.

KEY

▓ Palmar interossei (3)
▓ Lumbricals (4)
▓ Adductor pollicis
▓ Flexor digiti minimi brevis

- **The Setup:** You can do this stretch in any position: standing, sitting, kneeling—even lying down. You use one hand to stretch the other.

  Turn your right hand palm up. The knuckles flex, that is, they make your fingers curl toward your palm. This stretch gently opens the fingers the opposite way, into extension. Lay the index finger of your left hand across all the fingers of your right hand, slightly below the point where your palm separates into your fingers. Your left index finger will be sitting in the little notch between your palm and your fingers. Line up the other fingers of your left hand next to your index finger. Depending on the length of your right fingers, you may not need to press with all of your left fingers.

  Place your left thumb across the knuckles on the back of your right hand. As you look at your stretch setup, your left thumb will be hidden underneath your hand.

- **The Stretch:** At the same time, gently push your left fingers down as you push your left thumb up. Look for the stretchy feeling on the inside of your right hand, both at the top of your palm and between each main knuckle and the next joint as the finger moves toward its tip. The area at the top of your hand is likely to turn a little pink. This means you are getting the fluids moving in your hand. Repeat the stretch on the other hand.

- **Enhance Your Flexibility:** Try little adjustments of your finger position, searching for the spot that will best give you the feeling of gentle stretch. Allow your right thumb to float free. (You can also figure out how to adapt this stretch to your thumb.)

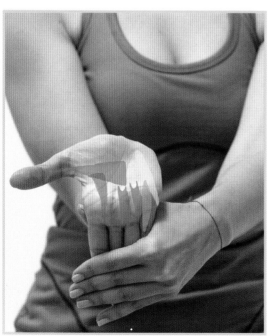

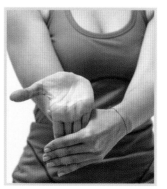

Note: For purposes of illustration, the Lumbrical shown here covers the right-most Palmar Interosseous.

34 hands: finger flexion

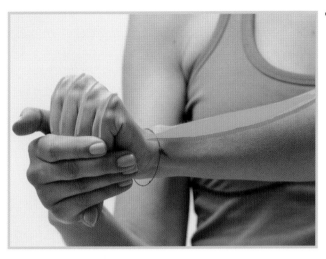

KEY

■ Extensor digitorum
■ Extensor digiti minimi

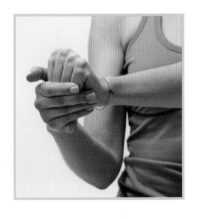

- **The Setup:** As in stretch 33, you can do this stretch in any position: standing, sitting, kneeling—even lying down. You use one hand to stretch the other.

  Look at the back of your left hand. There are three finger joints marked by knuckles: the one closest to the palm (main knuckle—1), the one halfway down your finger as you move toward the tip (2), and the one closest to the fingertip (3). Lay the index finger of your right hand across all the fingers of your left hand, between 1 and 2, very close to 2. Arrange the other fingers of your right hand in line next to the index finger. The fingers will spill over into the space between 2 and 3.

- **The Stretch:** At the same time, press your right fingers against your left fingers, and push back with the left fist. You are trying to push the fingers of your left hand closer to its palm. The fingers will begin to straighten. You will feel the stretch in your left fingers, in the space between 1 and 2. Repeat the stretch on the other hand.

- **Enhance Your Flexibility:** Experiment with placing your right thumb on the back of your left hand to increase the stretch feeling. Also, check on your left thumb. The stretch works best if the thumb is free of the right hand.

ENLIST YOUR MIND

This is not a common place to stretch, so it may take a few tries for your mind to register where your body is stretching. The technique is worth learning, because the full functioning of our hands is so important—both for everything we do in our life, and for our whole life long. It may help to close your eyes; push gently, one hand against the other; and reach with your mind into the fingers to discover the feeling of stretch.

Hips

In this section we will cover stretches for the hip flexors, the buttocks, and the side hip. The side-hip stretches—less commonly done—are particularly worth including in your quest for freely moving hips. Add to this group the inner thighs from the *Thighs* section (see p. 100), and you have a complete hip-opening sequence.

Causes of stiff, sore, or aching hip muscles/ muscles in spasm.	• Running or hiking along steep inclines or declines. • Sitting at a desk all day (or other long sitting session).
Injuries eased by stretching	• Lower-back muscle strain. • Lower-back ligament sprain (mild). • Piriformis syndrome. • Snapping hip syndrome (sometimes caused when your butt muscle "clicks" over your thigh bone).
Additional uses	• Before and after playing sports that use the hips a lot—such as cycling, golf, running, walking. • To protect your lumbar curve. If the external hip-rotator muscles become tight, they pull on the lower back and the lumbar curve flattens. Absent their natural curve, your lumbar discs are more likely to be compressed when you maintain a standing position. If you play sports, this problem is compounded. • To release tight "turnout" muscles. Although this book does not cover stretches for dancing, many people—especially women—studied classical ballet for a time as children. If you have this training, take a look at the habitual rotation of your leg, starting up at your hip. If your toes are positioned outside your heels, and this feels natural, you may have tight external hip rotators (the muscles that rotate your hip and toes out) and not realize it. Or, do you walk with "duck feet"? Stretch these muscles with stretches 38–40. (*Stretching* the external hip rotators and *strengthening* the internal hip rotators—the muscles that rotate your hip and toes in—will give you balance between the muscle groups.)

Pinpoint the area of discomfort (this connects your mind with your body), and choose the stretch that most closely reaches that spot.

For guidance on stretch duration, see pp. 32–33. To discover how to use breathing to deepen the stretch, see pp. 34–35.

35 hip flexors: knee-to-chest pull, supine

The following three stretches are a progression from least intense to most intense. If you are in pain or just beginning your flexibility training, experiment with stretch 35. When your body gets familiar with feeling the hip flexors stretching, you can add stretch 36, and finally stretch 37. Use the feeling in your body as your guide to how much stretch you can achieve on a particular day.

- **The Setup:** Lie on your back on a comfortable, supportive surface, with your legs at full length. Lace your fingers around your bent left knee and pull it to your chest, keeping the right leg straight. (You also have the option to pull behind your thigh, if pulling the knee feels uncomfortable.) Check your pelvis position. Make sure it is even—meaning that one pelvic bone is not lifted more toward the ceiling than the other, or more toward your shoulder than the other.

- **The Stretch:** Press your straight right leg to the floor while hugging your bent left knee to your chest. You will feel the stretch in the front of your right hip—where your hip bends when you lift your knee. Either hold the maximum position or gently press/pull and release in slow rhythm (see *Breathing,* p. 34). Repeat with a straight left leg and bent right knee.

- **Enhance Your Flexibility:** Stretch and point your toes. Make your straight leg even longer by sending your thigh and calf away from your torso. Your whole leg will come alive with vitality, creating more space in the front of the hip.

ENLIST YOUR MIND

Keep the back of your neck long—make sure your chin does not stick up toward the ceiling. Develop a strong mental connection with your body by gently reminding yourself to lengthen your neck. Soon you will find that your neck lengthens automatically.

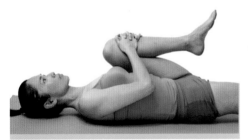

KEY

▐ Iliopsoas (psoas major and minor, iliacus)

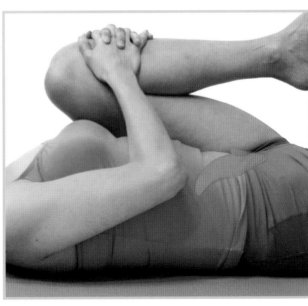

36 hip flexors: lunge, standing

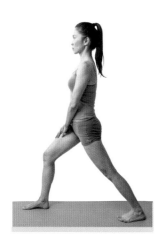

KEY

Iliopsoas (psoas major and minor, Iliacus)

Sartorius

Tensor fascia lata

Rectus femoris

- **The Setup:** Stand with your right leg forward and left leg behind you. Adjust the width of your stance for balance: if you need more stability, stand with your legs a little more apart. Toes should line up in front of heels—make sure they are not rotated outside your heels. Your front knee can be a little behind the ankle—just not in front of it. This protects your knee from strain. Hold your neck in a comfortable position—neither too lifted at the chin nor too bowed toward your chest. Just comfortable, without strain. Looking straight ahead helps to accomplish this.

  Your pelvic position is important here. Make sure your hip bones are even—top to bottom and front to back. (See "Enlist Your Mind," below.)

- **The Stretch:** Gently tuck your pelvis. The stretch will appear in the straight left leg—the back leg—at the hip-flexor level in front. At the same time, sense what's happening with your back leg: keep it straight. You can think: heel down, pelvis tucked. Repeat with right leg behind and straight, and left leg in front and bent.

- **Enhance Your Flexibility:** Experiment with what you feel when you send your front knee a little more forward toward your toes—a little more knee bend, then a little less. Just make sure your knee does not pass forward beyond your ankle.

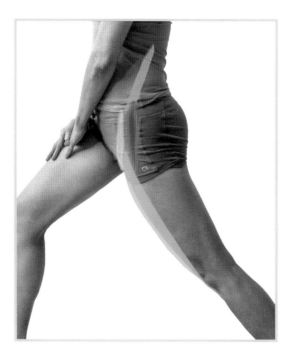

ENLIST YOUR MIND

Determine whether your pelvic bones are even in two ways. One bone should not lift more toward the ceiling than the other (level from top to bottom). One bone (usually on the bent-knee side) should not be more forward than the other (even from front to back).

You can use your front pelvic bones to guide you here. If you place your hands on your hips, middle fingers in front and thumbs in back, you will feel the iliac crest of the pelvic bone. If you follow the crest farther forward with your middle fingers, you can find a spot on the bone on each side to use as your marker of evenness.

37 hip flexors: lunge, kneeling

- **The Setup:** Kneel with your right leg forward and left leg behind you. Adjust the width of your stance for balance: for more stability, move your forward leg a little farther to the right. Your right toes should line up in front of your heel—make sure they are not rotated outside your heel. Your front knee can be a little behind the ankle—just not in front of it. This protects your knee from strain. For more support, kneel between two chairs, and place your hands on them if needed. Otherwise, place your hands lightly on your front thigh. Hold your neck in a comfortable position—neither too lifted at the chin nor too bowed toward your chest. Just comfortable, without strain. Looking straight ahead helps to accomplish this.

- **The Stretch:** Gently tuck your pelvis. The stretch will appear in the left leg—the back leg—at the hip-flexor level in front. When you experience the stretch in the right spot, you can intensify it by moving your front leg a little more forward. Ultimately, and with practice, your back hip will be much lower to the ground. On your way there, you will have moved your front foot forward in many small increments.

  Now comes an important point, which cannot be stressed enough. The hip-flexor stretch contains the beginning of a lovely back extension—also called an arch. Whenever we practice developing the back extension, we always encourage length: spine goes up as well as forward, to avoid scrunching the lower spinal vertebrae together. Repeat the stretch on the other side

- **Enhance Your Flexibility:** If you can connect with the feeling of lift in extension as you practice, you will begin to feel a deep abdominal stretch starting near the top of your kneeling leg. This is your iliopsoas group, which reaches deep into the interior of your body.

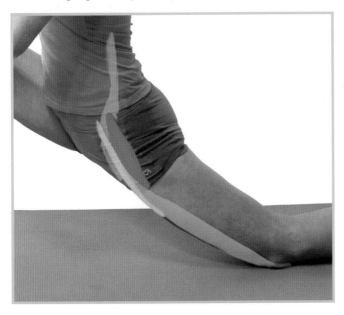

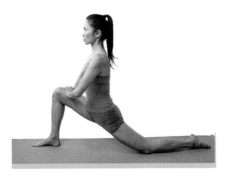

KEY

▮	Iliopsoas (psoas major and minor, Iliacus)
▮	Sartorius
▮	Tensor fascia lata
▮	Rectus femoris

38 buttocks: ankle crossed over knee, seated

- **The Setup:** Sit on a supportive chair (not an armchair) with your right foot on the floor and your left ankle crossed over your right knee. Adjust your left ankle so that it feels comfortable—make sure the ankle bone isn't digging into your thigh. Open your left knee out to the side.

- **The Stretch:** Lifting up your sacrum (pelvis) and lower back out of your hips, begin to lean slowly forward, keeping your back flat. The stretch will appear in the left side of your butt. The feeling in the muscles you are targeting for this stretch should be immediately obvious. A steady exhale–stretch/inhale–relax rhythm is a good tactic for this stretch. Repeat the stretch on the other side.

- **Enhance Your Flexibility:** When you're ready for more intensity, lean steadily forward without relaxing on your inhale. Keep your back as flat as you can. These two actions will develop intensity. Your goal is touching your chest to your thighs. Although you may not get there for a while, if you practice you will notice your chest getting definitely lower.

ENLIST YOUR MIND

On this one, your stretching mantra is: flat back, flat back. Think of lifting your pelvis up and away from the legs. Create lots of mental space in your hip joint, and soon there will be physical space there, making it easier to bring your torso up and forward.

KEY

- Inferior gemellus
- Obturator internus
- Superior gemellus
- Gluteus maximus

Note: The three deep hip-rotator muscles are actually located within the buttocks. For the purposes of illustration, we see them on the surface instead of deep inside and close to the pelvis.

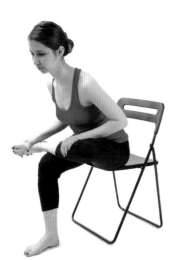

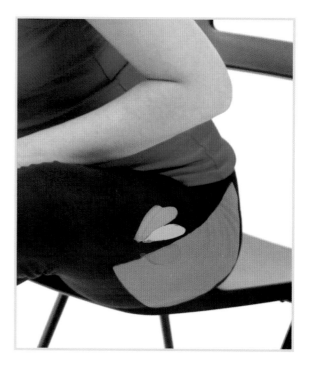

39 buttocks: cross-body lower-leg lift, supine

- **The Setup:** Lie on your back on the floor, using a carpet or mat if you want some cushioning. Stretch your legs straight out. Bend your right knee, open it out to the side, and hold your right ankle with your left hand. This is similar to the setup position in stretch 38, except that you are holding your right foot in your left hand instead of resting it on your left knee. Reach your left hand over or under your ankle—whichever position feels more comfortable. Right hand rests on the right knee.

- **The Stretch:** At the same time, pull your right ankle toward your chest and push your right knee away from it. You are trying to bring your right ankle to a position directly across from your right knee. Optimum position for this stretch is lower leg parallel to shoulder-girdle line. Look for the stretch in the right side of your butt. Repeat the stretch on the other side.

- **Enhance Your Flexibility:** When you first practice this stretch, it may be very tempting for your head to lift off the ground because your outside hip is so tight. You can certainly start this way, supporting your neck flexors by gently pressing your tongue to the roof of your mouth. After you spend some time in this stretch, and your body figures out what you are asking it to do, you will find your head gently releasing to the floor. Keep your left leg as straight as you can while stretching the right side of your butt.

ENLIST YOUR MIND

It is important to monitor the position of your neck. During the stage when you are working on settling your back to the floor, your neck will likewise lift. You don't want to introduce any extra tension or vertebrae scrunching in your neck, and one way to keep your neck relaxed while working on relaxing your back is to place a rolled-up towel behind your head, just opposite the bridge of your nose. Adjust the size of the towel depending on how far your neck lifts from the floor. Then check in with your mind: neck relaxes on the towel.

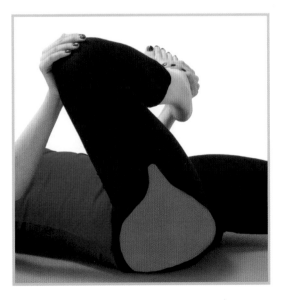

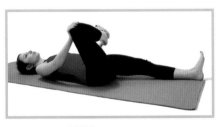

KEY
▇ Gluteus maximus

40 buttocks: crossed-knees foot pull, lying on back

ENLIST YOUR MIND

Use your mind to signal your neck to relax. It is especially easy here to allow your neck to shorten and your chin to point up. While you are holding the stretch, you might try cycling your mind through a short checklist several times. Check for the correct stretch position; then check for relaxation in the parts of your body that are not specifically receiving the stretch, that is, your neck.

- **The Setup:** Lie on your back on the floor, using a carpet or mat if you want some cushioning. Bend your knees and put your feet on the floor. Cross your left knee over your right, resting your left thigh on your right. (This is exactly the same thing you would do if you were sitting upright and wanted to cross your legs.)

- **The Stretch:** Lift your crossed knees toward your chest. Your right foot will be sticking out to the left, your left foot to the right. Reach up with your hands and grasp the outsides of your feet—right hand takes the left foot; left hand takes the right. Pull your feet farther out to the sides, away from each other. Repeat the stretch on the other side.

- **Enhance Your Flexibility:** This stretch sounds simple, but it requires more outside-hip flexibility than stretch 38, for example. You may want to prepare yourself with stretch 38 for a while before attempting this one.

  When you first get into this stretch position, you will feel a strong pull in the two sides of your butt. Your feet will not want to open, and your back may come off the floor. Your first task is to allow your back to sink back onto the floor—even before you increase the pull on your feet.

  Once you can sink your back to the floor, you can exert a little more pressure on your feet. You will gradually be able to move your hands from a position near your ankles to one farther along your feet toward your toes.

Note: All muscles shown are stretching on both sides of the body.

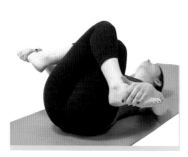

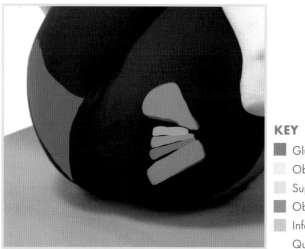

KEY

- Gluteus maximus
- Obturator externus
- Superior gemellus
- Obturator internus
- Inferior gemellus
- Quadratus femoris

41 side hip: knee push, lying on back

- **The Setup:** Lie on your back on the floor, using a carpet or mat to make you comfortable. Bend your knees and put your feet on the floor. Open your feet wider than your knees. Your knees remain in line with your hips, even though your feet are open.

- **The Stretch:** Drop your right knee inward, toward the floor. You should immediately feel a band of stretch around the outside of your right hip, beginning in your butt area and moving around to the side of your hip. Now cross your left knee over your right, and use the left knee to push the right gently toward the floor. Repeat the stretch on the other side.

- **Enhance Your Flexibility:** Stretching the side-hip area is not done as often as, for example, quadriceps and hamstrings, so it is likely that this stretch will be unfamiliar to your body. The main action here is allowing the knee to relax toward the floor, adjusting the pressure of the assisting leg as necessary. Whenever you feel the tightness in your right hip release a little, increasing the pressure from the assisting knee will increase your range of motion in this area.

ENLIST YOUR MIND

Here your work is primarily calming your mind's unease, since this stretch is both powerful and most likely new territory for your body. Sometimes a panicky feeling can arise with a powerful stretch, a feeling of "what if I break in half?!" Slow, deep breaths will help your body find a resting place within the discomfort of the stretch.

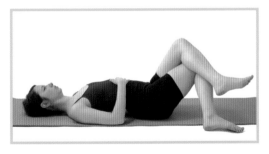

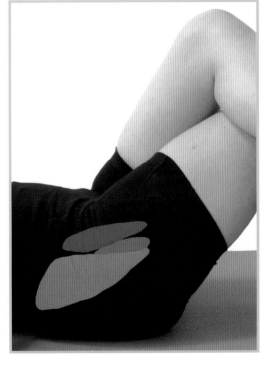

KEY
- Tensor fascia lata
- Gluteus minimus
- Gluteus medius

42 side hip: towel under hip, lying on side

- **The Setup:** Lie on your right side with your legs stretched out, one on top of the other. Place a rolled-up towel under your right hip. The placement of the towel is important: it goes between your pelvic bone (iliac crest) and your thigh bone (greater trochanter). Get familiar with both these bony landmarks on your side before you place the towel. You don't need to know anatomy: just feel the bones that come to the surface at your hip and thigh.

- **The Stretch:** The stretch appears in the side of your hip facing the ceiling. In other words, the towel lifts your bottom hip so you can experience greater range in the top hip. Gently brace yourself with the open palm of your left hand. You can rest your head either in your hand (elbow bent) or on your straight right arm. Repeat the stretch on the other side.

- **Enhance Your Flexibility:** For a greater stretch, use a larger towel. When you reach the point at which the world's largest towel still does not give you enough stretch because of the way it gives, try a rolled-up fitness mat or soft roller, which will elevate your hip higher. This is not necessary, however. At least at the beginning, the towel will work well.

ENLIST YOUR MIND

The trick here is to allow your abdominal and rib area to fall into the floor above the towel, and your thigh to relax into the floor below it. Keep sending thought messages of relaxation to those areas; allow them to drape over the towel and solidly settle onto the floor. Also, think left pelvic bone moving away from left thigh bone—and lots of space along the curve of your left hip.

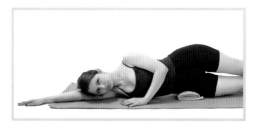

KEY

Tensor fascia lata
Gluteus medius
Gluteus minimus

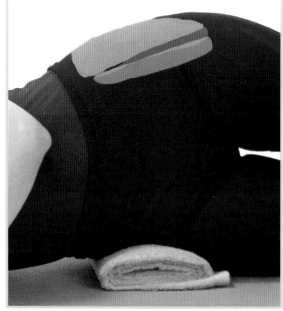

43 side hip: legs extending sideways, using arm

ENLIST YOUR MIND

ENLIST YOUR MIND

Connecting your mind to this stretch can be tricky. When you push your right hip toward the floor, at first you may feel your waistline stretching instead of the side of your hip. Be patient and keep working the hip gently toward the floor, searching for the feeling of stretch in a lower spot than the abdominals.

KEY

| | Quadratus lumborum
| | Tensor fascia lata
| | Gluteus medius

- **The Setup:** Lie on your right side at full length on the floor, using a mat or carpet to make you comfortable. Your legs are straight and stacked, one on top of the other. Lift your torso, keeping your head and shoulders in line with your legs and feet, and support yourself on your outstretched right arm. Make sure your right shoulder remains dropped and is not allowed to hike up.

- **The Stretch:** Gently push your right hip toward the floor. Without bending your arm, try to get the side of your hip flat against the floor. Of course this won't happen, but a stretch will happen instead. In the photo you see the left foot crossed in front of the right leg, and the left knee bent. Experiment with this position to see if it helps you push your hip toward the floor more easily. Repeat the stretch on the other side.

- **Enhance Your Flexibility:** Explore the balance between the distance of your hand from your body and your feeling of stretch. Adjusting the hand farther from or closer to your torso may enhance the feeling of stretch for you. This will be an individual adjustment for everyone.

  It is also important to keep your arm straight, but your shoulder dropped. This may take some practice. Many people have a tendency to bend the elbow when they try to drop the shoulder. You need the leverage that your straight arm will give you, but at the same time you must avoid sinking the neck into the shoulder.

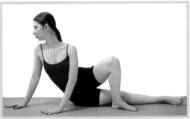

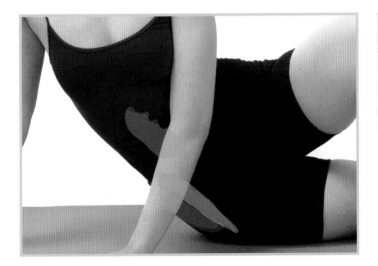

Note: In the illustration shown here, some of the muscles being stretched overlay the arm.

hips

99

PART TWO YOUR STRETCH REPERTORY

Thighs

This section presents stretches for the inner thighs/groin, quadriceps, and hamstrings. To feel thorough, all-around hip opening, choose stretches for all three areas and do them in the same session.

Causes of stiff, sore, or aching thigh muscles/ muscles in spasm	• Playing sports or doing activities that use repetitive leg movements—such as basketball, cycling, running, walking. • Any long sitting session—such as sitting at the computer or on an airplane flight.
Injuries eased by stretching	• Hip-flexor strain. • Iliopsoas tendonitis. • Quadriceps strain. • Quadriceps tendonitis. • Patellofemoral pain syndrome. • Patellar tendonitis. • Lower-back muscle strain. • Lower-back ligament sprain (mild). • Hamstring strain. • Piriformis syndrome. • Groin strain. • Tendonitis of the adductor muscles.
Additional uses	• Before and after playing sports or doing activities requiring constant thigh movement—such as basketball, cycling, running, walking. • Before and after playing sports or doing activities requiring use of the inner thighs for side-to-side movement—such as racquetball/handball. • To prevent hamstring tears in sports that require sprinting—such as racquetball/handball and running. • To increase thigh range of motion, which helps create larger strides for a sprint.

Pinpoint the area of discomfort (this connects your mind with your body), and choose the stretch that most closely reaches that spot.

For guidance on stretch duration, see pp. 32–33. To discover how to use breathing to deepen the stretch, see pp. 34–35.

44 inner thighs/groin: knees over hips, supine

This sequence of three stretches for the short adductors involves bending and opening the knees. It begins with a less intense stretch that can serve as a warm-up for the others (stretch 44). The second stretch changes the angle between knees and hips, shifting the focus of the pull (stretch 45). The third stretch adds intensity by using the body's weight to stretch the inner-thigh muscles (stretch 46).

- **The Setup:** Lie on your back on a comfortable surface, using a mat or carpet to cushion your spine. Bend your knees, keeping them together and placing your feet on the floor. Bring your knees toward your chest, placing them in line with your hips. The line should be straight from your hips to your knees—perpendicular to the floor.

    Placing one hand on each knee, open your knees to the side. Relax your heels against your butt.

- **The Stretch:** Gently press your knees open with your hands. You will feel the stretch along your inner thighs between knee and hip. Hold the position for a static stretch, or use a gentle push-out-on-exhale/release-slightly-on-inhale technique.

- **Enhance Your Flexibility:** There will be a limit to how much you can increase this stretch using your hands to aid you. Press your knees down with more force—but still gently.

ENLIST YOUR MIND

This is a stretch that uses the trainer-assisted-stretch concept. When a trainer passively stretches your muscles, your only job is to relax those muscles, breathe calmly, and allow the trainer's pressure to deepen the stretch for you. Your hands, arms, shoulders, and back now become stand-ins for the trainer. Make a separation in your mind between your upper body, which creates the stretch for you, and your inner thighs, which allow the stretch to happen. With practice, you will be able to relax some muscles and contract others.

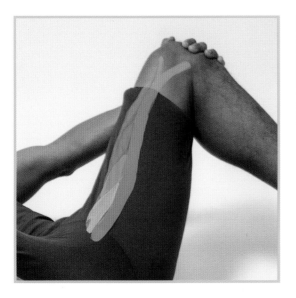

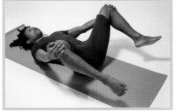

KEY

- Pectineus
- Adductor brevis
- Adductor longus
- Adductor magnus
- Gracilis

Note: All muscles shown are stretching on both sides of the body.

45 inner thighs/groin: feet on wall, supine

ENLIST YOUR MIND

This is a stretch in which your body is completely supported by the floor and the wall. You might try closing your eyes and imagining your knees opening wider. Pay attention to the feeling of stretch. As it gets less and you move your body closer to the wall, close your eyes again for a second round.

KEY

Pectineus
Adductor brevis
Adductor longus
Gracilis
Adductor magnus

- **The Setup:** Lie on your back on a comfortable surface, with a mat or carpet for support if you like, facing a wall. Bend your knees, with the soles of your feet together on the floor, right next to the wall. Crawl your feet up the wall and open your knees to the side. The outsides of your feet should now be touching the wall. Allow the outsides of your ankles to bend as you completely relax your feet against the wall.

- **The Stretch:** This is a passive stretch, which means you can let the position do the work for you while you concentrate on relaxing your muscles. Here the stretchy feeling is still in your inner thighs—but closer to your hip crease (groin) area. Keep breathing steadily and allowing your knees to continue to open.

- **Enhance Your Flexibility:** As you hold the position and your inner thighs relax and open more, try moving your body closer to the wall for a greater stretch. You will know the moment to do this, because the feeling of stretch recedes somewhat, allowing you to ask your body for more.

Note: In the illustration shown here, some of the leg muscles being stretched overlay the hand. All muscles shown are stretching on both sides of the body.

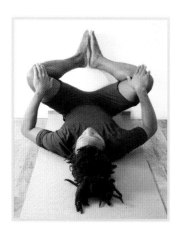

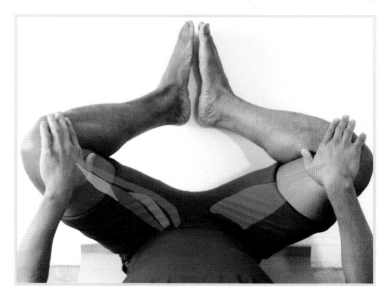

46 inner thighs/groin: hips over knees, prone

- **The Setup:** Kneel on the floor in an all-fours position, padding the floor for comfort if you like. Begin to open your knees slowly out to the sides. Line up your knees directly under your hips. When your knees are open as far as they will go, place your forearms on the floor and get as comfortable as you can in the position. Make sure your knees are in line with your hips—neither in front nor in back of them.

- **The Stretch:** As soon as you start opening your knees, you will feel the stretch in your inner thighs.

- **Enhance Your Flexibility:** This is the flip side of stretch 44, except that your weight is on top of the stretching muscles here, which makes this stretch more intense. Keep breathing regularly through the strong stretching feeling. You will be able to move your knees farther apart the longer you hold the stretch. Rock your butt a little behind your knees for a more intense feeling; then bring your knees back in line with your hips and see if you can move your knees farther apart.

ENLIST YOUR MIND

Imagine someone gently pressing on your sacrum/lower-back area, allowing your chest to come closer to the floor and your knees to separate more.

*Note: All muscles shown are stretching **on both sides** of the body.*

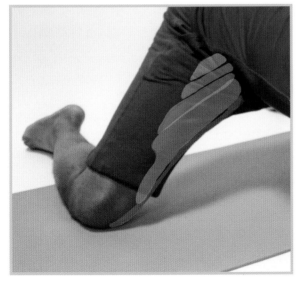

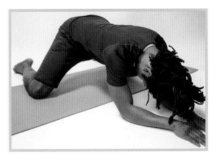

KEY

Pectineus
Adductor brevis
Adductor longus
Adductor magnus
Gracilis

47 inner thighs/groin: side lunge, standing

In the next two stretches the legs are straight and open, allowing access to the long adductor muscles, and complementing stretches 44–46 for complete inner-thigh flexibility.

- **The Setup:** Stand with your legs open wide enough to fit your shoulders between your heels. Bend your left knee and shift your weight to the left side. Place your hands on your left knee for stability. Allow your torso to bend forward as you push into your left thigh with your hands. Your right leg remains straight, with the foot anchored in place. (Instead of placing your hands on your knee, you can hold onto a stationary support, for example, a doorway or post.)

ENLIST YOUR MIND

Here you can experience the difference between an active and a passive stretch. Muscles in your left leg and hip are contracting, while muscles on the inside of your right leg are stretching. In this fairly simple stretch, with good strong support, your mind has a chance to sort out how it can pull off contracting and relaxing at the same time.

- **The Stretch:** The stretch will appear on the inside of your right leg as you lean toward the left side. To protect your left knee from injury, it is important to keep it lined up with the left toes: make sure it doesn't roll inwards. The placement of your right foot can be directly opposite or a little behind your left foot—whichever position you find more comfortable. Be careful not to move your foot too far back, or the stretch will shift to your hip-flexor area. Keep the stretchy feeling in your inner thighs. Repeat the stretch on the other side.

- **Enhance Your Flexibility:** Once you locate the feeling of stretch along the inside of your right leg, you can increase that feeling by adjusting your degree of torso lean. Experiment with leaning a little more forward, a little more upright. You will also get a greater stretch by pushing your left hip more to the left side, allowing your right leg to move closer to the floor.

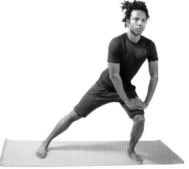

KEY

Pectineus
Adductor brevis
Adductor longus
Adductor magnus
Gracilis

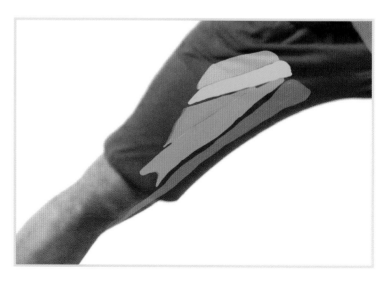

48 inner thighs/groin: straddle against wall

- **The Setup:** Sit with the side of your torso next to a wall. Push your thigh and butt right up against it. Then turn onto on your back and straighten your legs. Your butt and legs should end up right next to the wall and be supported by it.

- **The Stretch:** Slowly open your legs to the sides until you reach your maximum range of opening. You will feel a strong stretch in your inner thighs. Choose between bare feet or socks—whichever does not impede the further opening of your legs.

- **Enhance Your Flexibility:** Flex your feet, and activate both legs by lengthening through your heels. Now turn your toes a little toward the floor. This will rotate the muscles along the entire leg and produce a deeper stretch. Now breathe and relax your feet. This is a stretch—because of the comfortable lying position of your body—that lends itself to a static hold. Once your muscles get accustomed to how they feel in this position, you can stay in the stretch for two minutes, three minutes. Gradually increase the time.

KEY

■ Gracilis
□ Pectineus
■ Adductor brevis
■ Adductor longus
■ Adductor magnus

thighs

105

If your body really opened up for you, you must come out of the position slowly. If you shock your body, it may wish it hadn't opened. Try this method: place your hands one behind each thigh. Allowing your leg muscles to continue to relax, do all the work with your upper body. Pull behind the thighs so the knees bend a little. Push one leg over to meet the other (still without activating the leg muscles) as you roll over onto your side. Stay for a moment or so before you get up and move around.

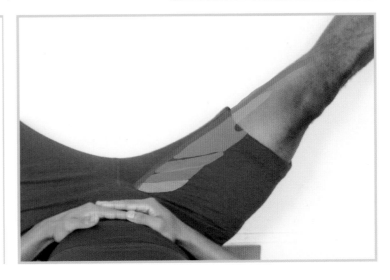

ENLIST YOUR MIND

This is a good stretch for closing your eyes, relaxing your legs as much as you can, and imagining your legs dropping more and more toward the floor. Then surprise yourself after your two-minute stretch and see how much closer to the floor they are.

Note: All muscles shown are stretching on both sides of the body.

49 quadriceps: heel to buttocks, prone

ENLIST YOUR MIND

You can get a subtle increase of stretch in this position by feeling into the front of your thigh with your mind. Take a couple of breaths to eliminate mental distractions. Imagine that your thigh is getting longer because it is separating from the hip joint and creating more space there. As you think this, gently send your right knee away from your right hip along the floor. If you are really tuned in to your muscles, you can feel greater space in the hip joint and greater stretch in the thigh.

KEY

Vastus lateralis

Rectus femoris

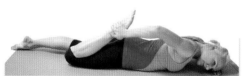

- **The Setup:** Lie face down on the floor, with your legs at full length. The stretch will involve one leg and one hand, so you can either rest your chin on the other hand, or turn your head sideways and rest your cheek on your hand.

- **The Stretch:** Reach back with your right hand and grasp your right foot. Slowly bring your heel in toward your butt. The stretchy feeling will appear in the front of your right thigh (which is resting against the floor). Gently press your hip bone to the floor, taking away any bend in your hip. The right side of your body is now a straight line from shoulder to knee.

  When you first practice this stretch, you may be unable to reach your foot with your hand. You can hook a towel around your foot (either small or large, depending on the length you need) so that you can still pull your foot toward your butt. With practice you will gain more range, and the towel will become unnecessary. The stretch is at its maximum when your knee touches your butt. Repeat the stretch on the other side.

  Make sure your legs are together. The knee of the stretching leg should be right next to the knee of the straight leg—not winging out to the side. Also, check that your foot comes straight toward the butt—not to the outside or inside of it. Correct alignment will make sure you have no joint problems as you practice.

- **Enhance Your Flexibility:** If you want a little extra flexibility challenge, adjust the position of your hand on your foot. Instead of placing it near your ankle, move your hand more toward your toes. This will add an extra dimension by also stretching the ankle and top of the foot.

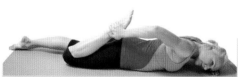

50 quadriceps: back shin on wall, kneeling

- **The Setup:** Kneel on the floor in front of a wall—supported by a carpet or a mat, if you like. Place your left foot in front with your knee over your ankle. Place your right knee as close to the wall as you can, with your right shin resting on the wall. Either place your hands on your left knee for support, or hold onto a piece of furniture or a wall. Keep your torso upright, and your shoulders and neck relaxed.

- **The Stretch:** As soon as you place yourself in the setup position, you will likely start feeling this stretch in the front of your right thigh. This is a powerful move with the ability to increase your range of motion quickly. Consequently, the effort involved is considerable. Breathe. Relax into the position as much as you can. Repeat the stretch on the other side.

- **Enhance Your Flexibility:** You are already asking your body for a great deal of flexibility here. In comparison to this stretch, stretch 49 is much less intense. Another place you will notice stretch is up the front of your right foot, which is resting against the wall.

  When you want to increase the stretching pull, gently tuck your pelvis and feel how the front-of-thigh stretch increases. Try a breathing rhythm: exhale/tuck your pelvis, inhale/release your pelvis.

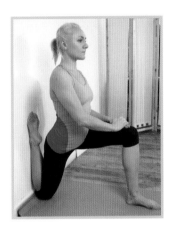

ENLIST YOUR MIND

The stretch here is likely to feel extreme. This is not a position that requires you to find the stretch—it will be quite evident. Use your mind to quiet your feeling of panic. Keep breathing and reassuring your body inwardly that it is okay, that it is safe to open up. If you can remain in the position for as long as a minute, you will find your body already responding to your mental signals, quieting down, and settling into the stretch a little more.

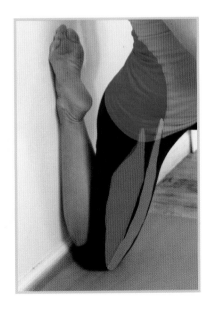

KEY

■ Vastus lateralis
■ Rectus femoris

51 hamstrings: one leg bent

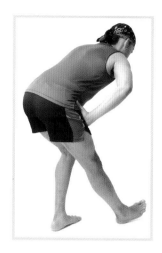

- **The Setup**: Stand with your feet about shoulder width apart. Bend your left knee slightly, and move your right foot out in front of the left to a comfortable distance. You should feel balanced. The position should be easy to hold. Flex your right (front) foot, and keep that leg straight. Your position is now: front leg straight, back leg bent.

  Place your palms on your right thigh, near your hip crease, and gently press. Make sure your pelvis is even.

- **The Stretch:** Keeping your back straight, begin to lower it slowly toward your thighs. You will feel the stretch in the back of the right (front) leg. Keep your neck curve in line with your spinal curve.

  Feel your way into this stretch. A long, slow pulse may work for you, or a static hold may be better. Once you become familiar with the position, you will be the best judge of what your body needs to allow it to expand its range of motion. There is some body weight leveraging the stretch; therefore, you can make this stretch more intense by leaning more weight forward. Always keep the back straight—"flat back" is the term used in fitness.

  Repeat the stretch with the left leg in front.

KEY

Semitendinosus

Semimembranosus

Biceps femoris (long head)

Biceps femoris (short head)

- **Enhance Your Flexibility:** What does an "even pelvis" mean? This term is often used, but perhaps not understood well. We want a level playing field from which to go into a stretch. You can locate your front pelvic bones just above your hip creases. When you perform this stretch, just make sure that the front pelvic bones are in line sideways. When someone does this stretch, it often happens that the straight front leg is allowed to pull the pelvic bone on that side forward. An even pelvis will always give you a better-aligned stretch.

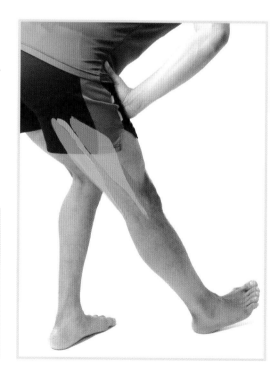

ENLIST YOUR MIND

Keep thinking: neck in line with spine; neck is long. It is common for people to crick their necks in this stretch. This will cause imbalance to your cervical vertebrae if done habitually. We want to be in a more ideal position after performing stretches—not introduce more things to fix. Remember: your view is your legs, not what's in front of you.

52 hamstrings: palms on floor, standing

- **The Setup:** Stand with your feet about shoulder width apart and shoulders relaxed. With your knees bent, roll your spine slowly downward, beginning at the top of your head, tucking your chin, and slowly rolling down through all your spinal vertebrae. When you pass your waist with your head, pull in your belly button to support your lower back as you continue to descend toward the floor. Stop when you are at the full extent of your present hip-flexion range. Your head and neck remain relaxed. Your view is of your own legs. You may already be feeling a stretch. Note how far your fingers are from the floor, so that you can compare their distance after you execute the stretch.

- **The Stretch:** Slowly straighten your legs. Take all the time you need. If you can straighten your legs without lifting your back up at the same time, you will achieve a deeper stretch. Here we emphasize stretch in the hamstrings. But keep in mind that, if your back is more in need of stretching, that is what you will feel. Any stretch that addresses the hamstrings will also lengthen the back. What you feel is determined by the area you most need to stretch.

- **Enhance Your Flexibility:**
  A variation of this stretch is to straighten first one leg and then the other, in a slow, alternating rhythm. Try the slow breathing rhythm: inhale/relax the knees; exhale/straighten one knee. As you allow one leg to relax when the knee bends, see if you can straighten the other leg without compensating by lifting your back. This will increase the stretch. Then try both legs together and see how much farther your fingers have progressed toward the floor.

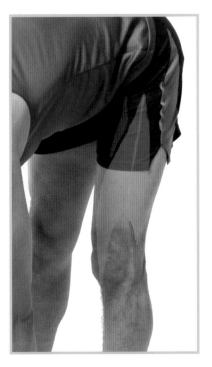

ENLIST YOUR MIND

When you reach your current lowest point in this stretch, make sure your legs are straight and your neck is relaxed. Close your eyes for 30 seconds. Either count slowly to 30, or set a 30-second digital alarm to free your mind. When you open your eyes, you may be surprised to find how much closer to the floor your head and hands are. Perhaps in some unconscious recess of your mind, you don't believe you can place your palms on the floor. Use this mind trick to change that belief. Your range will increase, and you will feel better.

Note: The muscles illustrated are on the back of the leg but, for the purposes of illustration, are shown on the front of the leg. All muscles shown are stretching on both sides of the body.

KEY

- Biceps femoris (long head)
- Biceps femoris (short head)
- Semimembranosus
- Semitendinosus

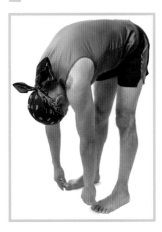

53 hamstrings: leg on raised surface, standing

ENLIST YOUR MIND

Keep developing your sense of lifting the back up and away from your legs. Visualize space in your hip joints to create this lift. Remember: your back is separate from your legs. It sounds obvious, but have you ever stopped to think that way when you stretch? Try this concept and see how your stretch range improves.

- **The Setup:** Stand on your left leg and lift your right leg onto a raised surface, such as a stool (your heel is near the stool's edge). To reach it more easily and get some extra support, slant your body relative to the stool. Move your left hip slightly left of the stool, allowing the right leg to rest slantwise on it. We are seeking even pelvic bones—side to side—to create the best angle for the stretch. So, when the right leg is up, check the pelvic-bone evenness. Locate your front pelvic bones by placing your hands on your hips, middle fingers in front and thumbs in back, to feel the iliac crest of the pelvic bone. Calculating your stance relative to your slantwise position, pull the right bone back so it is directly opposite the left one. Align your hips square to the direction you are facing—slantwise in this case. Now you're ready to stretch.

- **The Stretch:** As you lift your back straight up and away from your legs, lean slowly forward. Keep your back flat as long as you can. The stretch will develop in the back of your leg. When you can no longer keep your back straight and flat, allow it to curve forward, and bend to your fullest extent—today. Make sure your neck matches the curve of the rest of your spine, that is, keep your chin from jutting out. Repeat the stretch on the other side.

- **Enhance Your Flexibility:** On an exhale, flex your foot. As you inhale and relax it, try to bring your chest closer to your thighs. Repeat this inhale/exhale rhythm several times to increase your range. Another tactic is changing angles of the leg. Flex your foot and rotate your toes outward, away from the mid-line of your body. As you feel the increase in stretch in the back of your leg, try not to raise your back from its position. When you return the foot to its parallel position, see if you can lower your back still more. Spend some time coaxing more flexibility out of your leg.

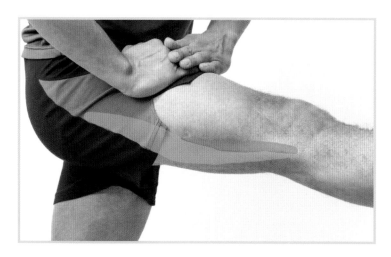

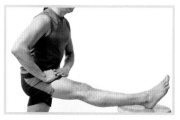

KEY
- Biceps femoris (short head)
- Biceps femoris (long head)

Calves

Silent and uncomplaining, the calves work behind the scenes in your life to allow you to pursue all your activities. These muscles will appreciate the tension release you can give them by stretching. (Note: the front of the calves is covered in the *Feet and Ankles* section—see p. 117.)

Causes of stiff, sore, or aching calf muscles/ muscles in spasm	• Walking down flights of stairs—such as exiting a high-rise building during an emergency. • Playing sports or doing activities that require a lot of lower-leg movement—basketball, cycling, racquetball/handball, running, swimming, walking. • Unfamiliar physical activities—calf muscles are especially affected by this. • Constant daily use. Since the lower leg supports the whole body, it carries the heaviest load when you walk or stand. Stretched muscles are less tense than tight ones, and can work harder and longer during your day.
Injuries eased by stretching	• Calf strain. • Achilles tendon strain. • Achilles tendonitis. • Medial shin splints (pain toward inside of shin). • Posterior tibial tendonitis.
Additional uses	• Before and after playing sports or doing activities requiring constant or intense lower-leg movement—basketball, cycling, racquetball/handball, running, swimming, walking. • During an aerobic workout to relieve calf tension and stress. • To prevent the cycle that results in soreness, tightness, cramping, restlessness, weakness—in the arch of the foot and calf muscles: Continuous support of whole body's weight → chronic use → muscle tightness and soreness → tendonitis and shin splints

Pinpoint the area of discomfort (this connects your mind with your body), and choose the stretch that most closely reaches that spot.

For guidance on stretch duration, see pp. 32–33. To discover how to use breathing to deepen the stretch, see pp. 34–35.

54a calves: heel flat on floor

The following three stretches—with front knee bent and back leg straight—take you along a continuum of intensity. All three use the same setup position. Stretch 54a is the basic stretch. Start with this one (a) if you are new to stretching; (b) if you are just getting warmed up for your session—whether flexibility, aerobic training, or weight training; or (c) if you are cooling down after an intense workout of another type—this is a time when your muscles need to start stretching gradually. Progress to stretches 54b and 54c when you feel ready for more intensity. The subtle adjustments in position that these stretches introduce will move you in stages along the road toward more freedom in your range of motion.

- **The Setup:** Stand facing a wall with your left foot forward and right foot back. Your left knee is bent; your back leg is straight. Place your hands on the wall for support at about shoulder height. Make sure your hip bones are even, that is, your pelvis is not rotated sideways in either direction. Place the heel of your right foot directly behind the toes: make sure the toes are not "winging" outside the heel.

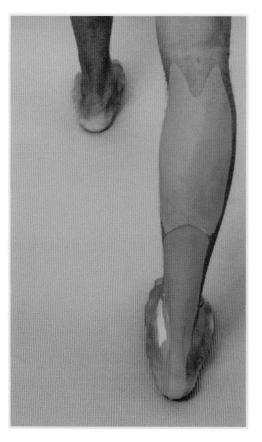

- **The Stretch:** Move your right foot gradually back, until it is as far back as you can move it without lifting your heel from the floor. You will feel this stretch in the "fat" part of your calf, below your knee. Repeat the stretch on the other side.

- **Enhance Your Flexibility:** As your body adjusts to the stretchy feeling in your calf, you will be able to move the heel farther back in small increments.

KEY

- ░ Gastrocnemius
- ▓ Achilles tendon
- Flexor digitorum longus
- ▓ Flexor hallucis longus

ENLIST YOUR MIND

Check on your head and general body posture. If you turn your head sideways and look into a mirror, you should see a straight line from the top of your head to your heel—no head drooping or butt sticking out.

54b calves: heel slightly raised

- **The Setup:** Start in the following position, described in stretch 54a. Stand facing a wall with your left foot forward and right foot back. Your left knee is bent; your back leg is straight. Place your hands on the wall for support at about shoulder height. Make sure your hip bones are even, that is, your pelvis is not rotated sideways in either direction. Place the heel of your right foot directly behind the toes: make sure the toes are not "winging" outside of the heel.

- **The Stretch:** Move your right foot gradually back, until it is as far back as you can move it without lifting your heel from the floor. Then, move your foot a little farther back, so that your heel comes off the floor. Press your heel down, but make sure that, no matter how much you press, your heel cannot touch the floor. You will feel this stretch in the "fat" part of your calf, below your knee. Repeat the stretch on the other side.

ENLIST YOUR MIND

Keep sending your heel into the floor, concentrating on feeling the stretch. Challenge your mind to see if you can keep the stretch in your awareness—to the exclusion of every other thought—for 30 seconds. Set a digital alarm to avoid asking your mind to count the seconds. It sounds simple, but you may find such single-minded concentration a challenge.

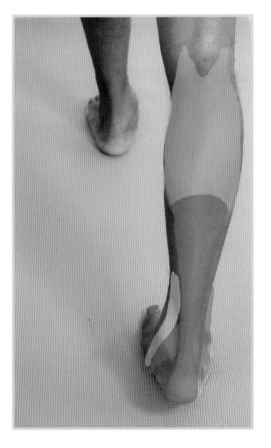

- **Enhance Your Flexibility:** As in stretch 54a, move your heel farther back in small increments as your body adjusts to the stretchy feeling in your calf.

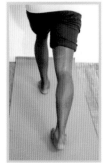

KEY

- Gastrocnemius
- Achilles tendon
- Flexor digitorum longus
- Flexor hallucis longus

54c calves: front knee moving slightly forward

ENLIST YOUR MIND

Bring your mind gently back to check on your alignment. Your head is in line with your neck, hips, and heels. Your body forms a slanted line from head to heel, without any bumps. It's always good to take a breath and relax your shoulders on the exhale. Shoulders often lift without our realizing it.

- **The Setup:** Start in the following position, used for stretches 54a and 54b. Stand facing a wall with your right foot forward and left foot back. Your right knee is bent; your left leg is straight. Place your hands on the wall for support at about shoulder height. Make sure your hip bones are even, that is, your pelvis is not rotated sideways in either direction. Place the heel of your left foot directly behind the toes: make sure the toes are not "winging" outside the heel.

- **The Stretch:** Move your left foot gradually back, until it is as far back as you can move it without lifting your heel from the floor. As in stretch 54a, you will feel this stretch in the "fat" part of your calf, below your knee. Concentrating on the feeling of stretch in your calf, begin to move your right knee slowly forward. You will feel an increase in stretching intensity. Repeat the stretch on the other side.

- **Enhance Your Flexibility:** Experiment with pushing the intensity limit by moving your left heel a little farther back so that it cannot touch the floor, as in stretch 54b. You have now introduced two extra levels of intensity: your right knee slightly more forward, and your left heel slightly farther back—reaching for the floor but not quite touching it.

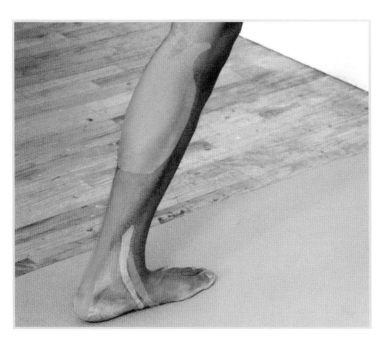

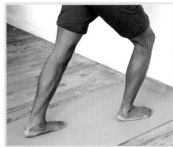

KEY

Gastrocnemius
Achilles tendon
Flexor digitorum longus
Flexor hallucis longus
Tibialis posterior

55a calves: ball of foot supported, leg straight

These two stretches involve dropping your heel down off a stable support. The first stretch (leg straight) primarily addresses your upper calf. The second stretch (knee bent) lengthens the lower calf.

- **The Setup:** Stand on a step with your hand on a support—the stair railing if you are on a flight of steps. Place your feet about shoulder width apart. Hang your right heel off the step, placing your weight on your left foot for balance. The ball of your right foot should be securely on the step. Find a spot somewhere in the middle of your right foot—not too far forward or back—where your foot feels stable, and yet your heel can hang comfortably off the step. Keep your right leg straight.

- **The Stretch:** Slowly allow your right heel to sink more and more off the step. The stretch appears in the "fat" part of your calf. Repeat the stretch on the other side.

- **Enhance Your Flexibility:** Increase the intensity of this stretch by adding more of your body's weight to your right heel as it sinks down off the step. You may feel the front of your right ankle resisting as your heel sinks lower. It may not be used to creating this degree of bend. That is okay—just keep breathing and allowing your ankle to relax.

ENLIST YOUR MIND

Increasing the intensity in this way can be subtly scary. As you shift more of your body's weight onto your stretching side, you may feel less secure on your supporting side. Just remind yourself that, at any moment, in a flash you can shift your weight back onto the supporting foot, should you feel in any way insecure in your stance.

KEY

- ◼ Flexor digitorum longus
-   Tibialis posterior
- ◼ Flexor hallucis longus

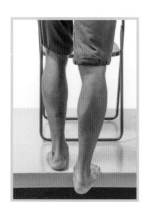

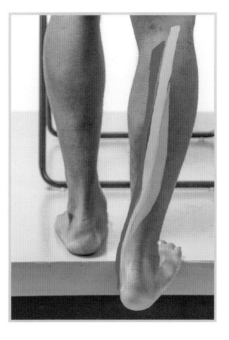

calves

PART TWO YOUR STRETCH REPERTORY

55b calves: ball of foot supported, knee bent

- **The Setup:** Stand on a step with your hand on a support, as in stretch 55a. Your feet are about shoulder width apart. Your left heel hangs off the step, with your weight on your right foot. Find a secure spot on the ball of your left foot where your foot feels stable as you hang your heel comfortably off the step. At this point your left leg is straight.

- **The Stretch:** Slowly sink your left heel down off the step, as in stretch 55a. Now gently bend your left knee, while still sinking your left heel down as far as you can. The stretch is still in your calf, but it now shifts to the lower part, nearer to the ankle and Achilles tendon. Repeat the stretch on the other side.

- **Enhance Your Flexibility:** The intensity of this stretch increases when you sink your heel more heavily, as in stretch 55a. If you feel the front of your left ankle resisting when you allow your heel to sink lower, try reinforcing the feeling that all your weight is on your right foot. You want to create a safe feeling for your body, so it feels that it can open in the way you're asking. Keep breathing always— slow, calm breaths go a long way toward creating your body's safe place.

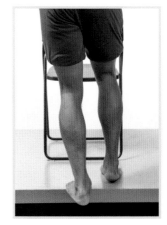

KEY

Soleus
Achilles tendon
Flexor hallucis longus

ENLIST YOUR MIND

Feeling this stretch—and therefore increasing your range of motion—require connecting your mind to your lower calf. It sounds unlikely, but your body may be feeling the stretch "behind the scenes," while "you" are prevented from feeling it because your mind is disconnected from the area you're stretching. That goes for stretches in general, but here is a good place to use some connection-increasing strategies.

To enhance your mental connection with your body in this stretch, try the following:

- Switch to a different stretch for the lower calf/Achilles tendon. For example, kneel on the floor with your left knee, and place your right foot on the floor next to it. Your right knee will be very close to your chin. Just lean forward and look for the stretch in your right lower calf. After you try a different stretch, your body may develop more awareness in the area you're targeting.
- Massage the Achilles tendon area with olive oil and/or a few drops of essential oil such as lavender. Stimulating the area will bring your body's awareness to it.

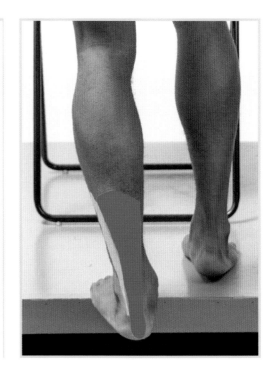

Feet and ankles

This section introduces stretches for the toes and ankles (including the front of the calves). Feet and ankles can really benefit from any stretching attention you give them. Our feet are too often encased in stiff or tight shoes, eventually reducing their ability to move freely. Here is a chance to regain and increase their flexibility.

Causes of stiff, sore, or aching foot and ankle muscles/ muscles in spasm	• Playing sports or doing activities requiring constant foot movement—such as basketball, cycling, racquetball/handball, running, swimming, walking. • Long periods of standing.
Injuries eased by stretching	• Ankle sprain (mild). • Anterior shin splints (pain toward outside of shin). • Flexor tendonitis. • Peroneal tendonitis. • Posterior tibial tendonitis. • Plantar fasciitis.
Additional uses	• Before and after playing sports or doing activities requiring constant foot movement—basketball, cycling, racquetball/handball, running, swimming, walking. (**Note:** almost any sport you can name will benefit from flexible feet. Even swimming: though your feet are not supporting your weight, if they can flex and bend freely as they travel through the resistive water medium, they become "flexible flippers." You will feel your foot muscles working.) • To prevent twisted ankles (stretch 59). • To keep your ankles flexible and improve their movement range—both for athletic activities (stretches 58 and 59). • To improve stamina—stronger cardiovascular capabilities. • To lower the risk of leg strain and pain during exercise.

Pinpoint the area of discomfort (this connects your mind with your body), and choose the stretch that most closely reaches that spot.

For guidance on stretch duration, see pp. 32–33. To discover how to use breathing to deepen the stretch, see pp. 34–35.

56 feet: standing toe flexion

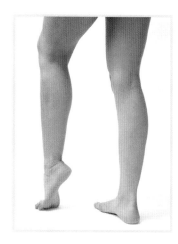

- **The Setup:** Stand next to a wall, a table, etc., so you have solid balance support available. The surface you stand on should be comfortable when you press your bare feet against it. You can use a thick mat or a carpet.

- **The Stretch:** Lift your left heel so your foot bends at the ball of the foot. Your knee remains bent for this stretch. Lean your knee and the front of your foot forward, increasing the angle of bend between your toes and the rest of your foot. Keep your toes flat on the floor. You will feel the stretch in the toes, across the metatarsal arch (underside of the toe knuckles), and sometimes even up into the sole of the foot. Repeat the stretch on the other side.

- **Enhance Your Flexibility:** This stretch requires time and practice to gain foot flexibility like this. Many people start out with hardly any bend-ability at all. When you get a 90-degree angle between your toes and the rest of your foot, that is a large landmark, an indicator of great progress. It is possible to gain more flexibility than 90 degrees—the more you lean your knee and front of your foot forward, the greater the stretch feeling, and the greater the potential for increased range.

KEY

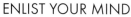 Flexor hallucis longus
Flexor digitorum longus
Abductor digiti minimi
Flexor digitorum brevis

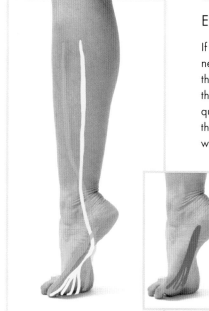

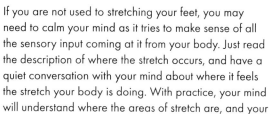

ENLIST YOUR MIND

If you are not used to stretching your feet, you may need to calm your mind as it tries to make sense of all the sensory input coming at it from your body. Just read the description of where the stretch occurs, and have a quiet conversation with your mind about where it feels the stretch your body is doing. With practice, your mind will understand where the areas of stretch are, and your focus will become sharper. Then your practice will become more efficient: you will laser in on the feeling of stretch from the first moment you place your body in the right position.

57 feet: standing toe extension

- **The Setup:** Stand next to a wall, a table, etc. (as in stretch 56), so you have solid balance support available. You will be working with the bony top-knuckle surfaces of your toes, so use a mat or carpet to make you comfortable when you press your bare feet against it.

- **The Stretch:** Lift your right heel and, without placing any weight on your toes, place the tips of your toes on the floor, perpendicular to it. Now, roll your toes forward and gently press them into the floor. The stretch appears on the top of your foot, especially in your toes. Repeat the stretch on the other side.

- **Enhance Your Flexibility:** Allow your toes to be long, without tension—uncurled along the floor. You can go two ways with this stretch. You can concentrate mostly on your toes, and back the rest of the foot off—in other words, create a bend in the foot near the toes (not something many people are familiar with). Or, you can gently push your right heel more and more forward to stretch the whole front arch of your foot, and up into your ankle.

ENLIST YOUR MIND

An important task for your mind on this stretch is stretching all the toes evenly. Our ankles are much more flexible on the outer side than on the inner (the "turned ankle"). Check that you are not pushing the foot to the outside—"sickling" the foot. Keep all the toes rolling straight forward for an even, across-the-foot stretch.

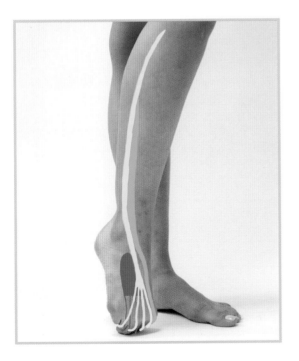

KEY

- Extensor digitorum longus
- Extensor digitorum brevis
- Extensor hallucis longus

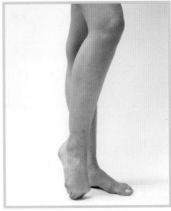

58 ankles: seated extension, using towel

ENLIST YOUR MIND

When you hold this stretch for 30 seconds to a minute, it is possible your mind will fight with you. It is simply challenging to work on a stretch like this, and your mind may be squirming and begging off. It can help to use a stopwatch, to breathe slowly and deeply, and/or to assure your mind that "it will soon be over."

- **The Setup:** Sit on your heels with a rolled-up towel under your flat feet. The tops of your feet rest on the towel. Place your toes up on the towel, and let the rest of your foot drape off it onto the floor.

- **The Stretch:** The setup already places your feet in the stretch. You will feel it above the toes, moving toward the ankle. No need to repeat on the other side: this stretch does both feet at once.

- **Enhance Your Flexibility:** The sitting position of this stretch requires that your quadriceps (front of your thighs) are stretched first. Otherwise, your butt will not reach your heels when you attempt to sit on them. (Use stretches 49 and 50 for this.)

  When you are ready for more stretch in the top of your foot and ankle, either: use a larger towel; or adjust the position of your toes on the towel—bring them farther forward to increase the arc of your foot.

KEY

Extensor digitorum longus

Note: All muscles shown are stretching on both sides of the body. The muscles being stretched are on the front of the foot.

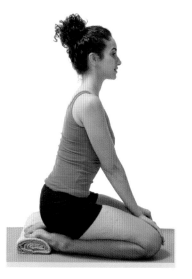

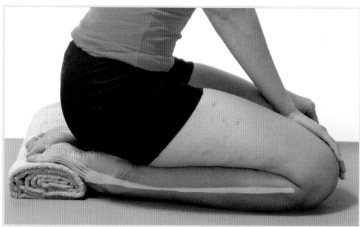

59 ankles: seated inversion, foot over knee

- **The Setup:** Sit either on the floor or on a supportive chair (not a cushy one—you don't want to sink in). On the floor, extend your right leg straight out in front of you. Cross your left ankle over your right knee. In a chair, your right foot will be on the floor. Cross your left ankle over your right knee.

- **The Stretch:** Rest your left foot comfortably on your right thigh, and allow your left ankle to bend in its natural direction—toward the outside of the foot. You will feel the stretch all around the outside of the ankle. This is a milder form of "turning the ankle"—same motion, just without the suddenness and violence. Repeat the stretch on the other side.

- **Enhance Your Flexibility:** The more securely your left foot rests on your right thigh, the more your body will relax and allow maximum stretch of the outside ankle. Take a breath. As you exhale, melt all resistance away: let your body sink the ankle into the stretch with confidence.

ENLIST YOUR MIND

Here's some information for your mind to digest: This is a nice, simple way to ensure that, in the event you have an ankle-turning episode, no swelling or tenderness will occur. The more range your ankle has, the less likely it is that injury will result. Since this can happen to anyone—a misjudged kerb on a dimly lit street, a lack of attention at the wrong moment—doing this stretch is real injury prevention.

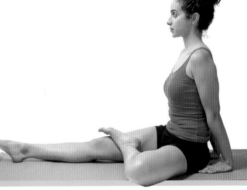

Note: The muscles stretching are on the outside of the calf but, for the purposes of illustration, are shown on the inside of the calf.

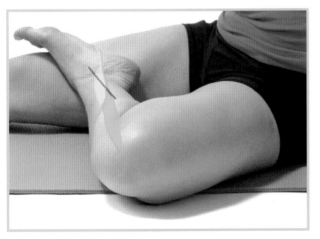

KEY
- Peroneus longus
- Peroneus brevis
- Peroneus tertius

Compound stretches

In this section we explore some very special stretches, which target more than one area at a time. When you feel ready to embark on these compound stretches, you are entering the realm of advanced stretching.

Before you start

When you practice this series of stretches, your understanding of flexibility training will take a quantum leap. Although the body, in fact, cannot really stretch any muscle to the exclusion of all others, it is usual to take the approach of targeting a specific muscle group with stretches that *emphasize* that group. The stretching feeling is therefore primarily felt in that group, for example, hamstrings or lower back. This is the approach mostly followed in this book.

But in reality there is much more going on in the body when a specific stretch is done, and in using an isolation approach we can forget that our bodies do not really stretch that way.

I hope that the explanations provided for the three following stretches will allow you to expand your concept of how your body stretches—giving you a springboard of understanding from which you can move ahead quickly in your flexibility training.

Benefits conferred by doing each stretch are listed separately in the sections that discuss the body areas each stretch addresses. For a listing of situations in which the stretches in this section can be useful, consult the pages, right, for each body area addressed.

Pinpoint the area of discomfort (this connects your mind with your body), and choose the stretch that most closely reaches that spot.

For guidance on stretch duration, see pp. 32–33. To discover how to use breathing to deepen the stretch, see pp. 34–35.

Injuries and Other Situations Helped by Stretching Muscles Involved in:

Forward Bend	Lower Back	(see p. 58)
	Hamstrings	(see p. 100)
The Plough	Lower Back	(see p. 58)
	Hamstrings	(see p. 100)
Seated Straddle	Lower Back	(see p. 58)
	Hamstrings	(see p. 100)
	Inner Thighs	(see p. 100)

During each technique, look for the feeling of stretch in the areas described.

THE MELT® METHOD

You may have upper-back curvature that causes your head to be carried too far forward of the shoulders when you are standing. If so, when you lie down to stretch on your back, the back of your neck will compress and your chin point toward the ceiling. To remedy this imbalance, consider The MELT® Method upper-body length and compression techniques.

The extreme version of this forward head carriage is called "dowager's hump." The hump is extra tissue created as the body attempts to balance the extra weight of the head, which is being carried farther forward than its natural structure allows. If you need a towel under the back of your head when you stretch on your back to prevent your neck from shortening, investigating the techniques of The MELT® Method is a good idea. You definitely want to reverse this condition, and prevent it from progressing. (See *Further Study*, p. 185, for more information.)

60 forward bend

- **The Preparation:** This stretch primarily targets your lower back/sacrum and hamstrings. The following stretches will prepare your body for it:
  a   Lower Back: stretches 11–17.
  b   Hamstrings: stretches 51–53.
  c   Full Spine: stretches 22–24 (for extra back preparation).

- **The Setup:** Sit on the floor with your legs extended in front of you, on a carpet or mat if you like. Make sure you are (relatively) comfortable. When you first begin to practice, it may, of course, be uncomfortable for you to sit on the floor in this position.

- **The Stretch:** Lifting your lower back away from your hips, stretch your torso up and forward toward your thighs. You will feel the stretch in your lower back/sacrum, and in your hamstrings (back of your legs).

- **Enhance Your Flexibility:** When you perform compound stretches, you will feel the most tightness in the muscle group you need to stretch the most. If, when you go into your forward bend, you have stretched your hamstrings but not your lower back/sacrum, you will likely feel most stretch in your lower back. Ditto for your hamstrings.

  So, with that knowledge, try picking one lower-back stretch and one hamstring stretch for your preparation. Spend some time in each before you go into your forward bend. Experiment with some different breathing methods. Then try your forward bend. Notice how far you can stretch, and where you feel the stretch. If you do this consistently when you practice—perhaps trying a different pair of stretches each time for a while—you will start to identify what your body prefers as a preparation stretch. Ask yourself what stretches bring your head closest to your thighs in the forward bend.

ENLIST YOUR MIND

Very important here is your mental connection to the feeling of lifting your lower back/sacrum away from your hips. Once you get the idea of how this feels, there will be more space in the hip joint, more freedom for your lower back to move up and away from your hips. Voilà! You move farther forward.

KEY

Erector spinae:
- Iliocostalis
- Longissimus thoracis
- Spinalis thoracis

- Biceps femoris (long head)
- Biceps femoris (short head)

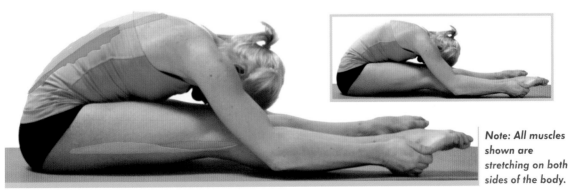

Note: All muscles shown are stretching on both sides of the body.

61 the plough

- **The Preparation:** This stretch primarily targets your lower back/sacrum and hamstrings (as in stretch 60). Use the following stretches to prepare your body for doing it:
  a Lower Back: stretches 11 – 17. Stretch 11c is a version of The Plough as well, Stage 3 in a gradual progression of stretches. If you can already perform a plough easily, use the information in this section to increase your understanding of it.
  b Hamstrings: stretches 51 – 53.
  c Full Spine: stretches 22 – 24 (for extra back preparation).

- **The Setup:** Lie on your back on the floor, using a mat or carpet for comfort if you like. Bend your knees and place your feet on the floor. (For entry method "c" below, your legs will be straight.) Arms are by your sides, palms down.

- **The Stretch:** There are several ways to enter the plough position. Use whichever one matches your flexibility level on the day you stretch. Our bodies are different from day to day. As you practice stretching, you will get to know your general flexibility level, and learn to recognize when you are a little under your usual bar, and when you are really sharp.

  Try these ways to enter the plough:

  a In stages: use stretches 11a, b, and c as steps to get into your full plough.
  b Core-assisted, bent knees: combining a gentle hand push to your butt with a pull of your core musculature, pull your knees up and over your head.
  c Core-unassisted, bent knees: once your core becomes strong from performing other elements in your fitness program, eliminate the hand push and use your core musculature solo to pull your knees up and over your head.
  d Core-unassisted, straight legs: in this method you combine your mastery of strength and flexibility by stretching your legs through your toes, contracting your core and, without arching your ribs, lifting your legs straight up and over your head.

  Once you get your legs over your head, you may find them trying to roll down again. This is okay. It means your back is not yet stretched enough for the weight of your legs to hold it over your head. Maintain a gentle pressure with your hands to keep your butt and legs in their

ENLIST YOUR MIND

For maximum experience of the plough, ask your mind to locate the muscle groups that need supplementary stretching before you do this challenging pose. This is not especially elusive. Just form the thought: does my back feel stiff? The backs of my legs? And you will know where you need to concentrate when you prepare to do the plough.

SAFETY NOTE

This is a demanding stretch. Make sure your body is adequately prepared to undertake it: perhaps even enlist an experienced instructor to guide you. Attempting this position too quickly can result in injury and set your progress back. Patience during the learning phase will give you a solid skill for the rest of your life.

FINE-TUNING—CALVES

After you have been practicing the plough for a while, you will get to an advanced stage of connection between your mind and your body. Translation: which muscle groups are keeping you from the full experience of the stretch? Calves may be one of these places. Limber up your calves using stretches 54 and 55.

position. This is a training stage—soon your back will be open enough to hold the position, and you will be able to release your hands.

If you have never been able to pull off a plough, the first time you do one is cause for elation. This stretch is a milestone in your flexibility progress. Being able to perform it—even once—shows off your ability to stretch several muscle groups at once. Breathe in the stretch; ask your body to relax.

Hold the position only as long as you feel comfortable. Dismount from the plough while you can still control the movement of your body. You want to avoid a *splat* dismount, that is, an out-of-control, not-sure-where-you'll-land situation.

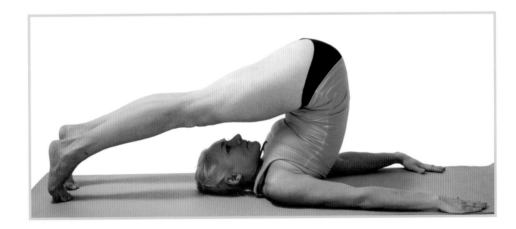

KEY

▮ Semimembranosus
▮ Semitendinosus
▮ Biceps femoris (long head)
▮ Biceps femoris (short head)

Erector spinae:
▮ Iliocostalis
▮ Longissimus thoracis
▮ Spinalis thoracis

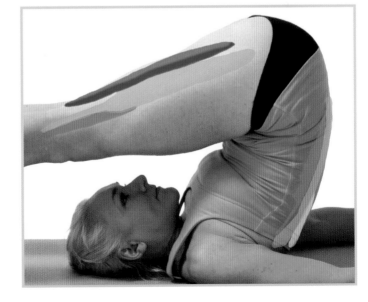

Note: All muscles shown are stretching on both sides of the body.

Come out of the stretch in one of several ways:

a   As in stretches 11a, b, and c: slowly bend your knees again and return, through stretch 11b, to your original position with knees to chest.

b   Hand-assisted: press your palms down onto the floor to help your core bring your legs back from over your head. Use your hands to control your back's descent to the floor. When your back is on the floor again, either bend your knees and hug them to your chest, or challenge your core by slowly bringing your straight legs down to the floor (without lifting your ribs as you lower them).

c   Core only, arms overhead: even if your core is already quite strong, you may still not be able to pull this off without your hands. This is because you still need a little more flexibility in your back, to complement your core strength. When you gain both of these elements, you will experience pinpoint control of both the back-roll-down and the leg-lowering phases.

d   Core only, arms by your sides: this is the most challenging dismount method. All the comments in "c" above apply. When you can dismount with your hands by your sides, your core is very strong.

Once you are able to extend your legs fully over your head, you are ready for the refinements. See "Enhance Your Flexibility," below.

- **Enhance Your Flexibility:** This is a many-faceted pose. Here are three tips:

a   Use the weight of your legs: when you first succeed in straightening your legs and taking them over your head, it is likely that your feet will not reach the ground. This is okay. This, too, is a stage in your practice—it cannot last in the face of gentle, persistent training. Just getting your legs over your head is a huge victory. As you allow them to hang off the floor, their weight will pull your back into a greater stretch.

b   Protect your neck: you may notice that your neck feels scrunched. Indeed, this is why some fitness books advise you to steer clear of this stretch. But you can develop awareness of your upper back and allow it to drop toward the floor, thus allowing your neck vertebrae to remain long—and safe from injury. (To develop upper-back flexibility, work on stretches 18–21.)

c   Toes on floor: when your toes start to touch the floor behind you, you are gaining more flexibility in your hamstrings. Gradually, if you continue practicing this stretch, you will be able to place the full length of your toes on the floor, and actually rock your body back and forth, feeling the stretch change between hamstrings and back, hamstrings and back. This is an advanced stage of success.

62 seated straddle

- **The Preparation:** This stretch primarily targets your lower back/sacrum, hamstrings, and inner thighs. The following stretches will prepare your body for it:
  a Lower Back: stretches 11 – 17.
  b Hamstrings: stretches 51 – 53.
  c Inner Thighs: stretches 44 – 48.
  d Full Spine: stretches 22 – 24 (for extra back preparation).

- **The Setup:** Sit on the floor, on a carpet or mat—whatever makes you comfortable. You are going into a demanding position and you do not want to be distracted by hard bones against the floor. Open your legs as wide as you can. This is your opening position.

- **The Stretch:** Slowly, lift your torso up and out of your hips and allow it to bend forward. Keep your back flat for as long as you can. When you are at your peak lower-back range, you can allow your back to round as you go forward as far as you can.

- **Enhance Your Flexibility:** Here, a key consideration is creating space in your hip joints. As you imagine space in the joint that allows your legs to pull away from your hips, you might actually use your hands to lift each leg out and away from your hip. Perhaps repeat this action a couple of times to help your body get the idea. If there is more space in your hip joint, your lower back will be able to lift up and away more easily. Each little thing you do to help your body settle into the stretch makes an imprint on it that contributes to more range over time.

ENLIST YOUR MIND

Make sure your shoulders are relaxed. Allow your head to drop forward and add its weight to the pull on your back. Your head weighs between 8 and 10 lb (3.5 and 4.5 kg)—the weight of a small bowling ball. Think of your head as the ball at the end of a ball-and-chain apparatus. Each link in the chain is a vertebra in your back. If you have prepared your back properly, none of the links will be stuck together. They will be free enough so that each of them can feel the effect of the ball at the end of the chain—dragging them forward and down.

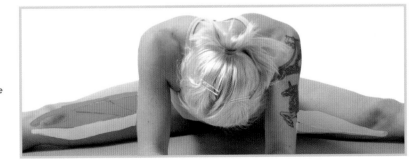

KEY

- ▓ Adductor longus
- ▓ Adductor brevis
- ▢ Gracilis
- ▓ Adductor magnus
- ▢ Semimembranosus
- ▢ Semitendinosus

Note: Muscles on the left leg are stretching on the back of the leg. For the purposes of illustration, they are shown on the front of the leg. All muscles shown are stretching on both sides of the body.

The next level

In this section we will introduce and begin to explore the split and the back bend, two very challenging techniques. These stretches are very different from all the others in this book. When you study how to perform the split and back bend, you are making a transition from basic to advanced stretching. This is truly "playing with the big boys."

Before you start

Developing the extreme flexibility that enables you to do a split and a back bend is, of course, by no means necessary to the lives of most of us—that is, it is not required for health and ease of living in the same way we need enough back and hamstring flexibility to be able to bend over and touch the floor. We might need to pick up something off the floor in the course of a day, but we will probably not need to push ourselves straight up from the floor with our stomach facing the ceiling.

I include these stretches in this book as a challenge. In my own training, the split and the back bend have always had an air of mystery about them. People could do them—or they couldn't. But detailed instructions, practical steps for how to make these moves possible, have been pretty thin on the ground. I want to save you the trouble of the big search I did. Therefore, I think it important to set forth a concrete plan that anyone who wishes can implement—and end up being able to do a split and/or a back bend.

The good news is that splits and back bends are quite attainable. They do not have to be mysterious and out of reach for the "normal" person. They do not have to be dangerous. Like any other branch of physical expertise, if you train correctly, you can attain the object.

Consistent effort is the key. You will not go all the way down in a split tomorrow just by reading about how to get there. You have to put in the time. But, for those of you who like a challenge, a goal to inspire you to work on your flexibility, learning these stretches is a project worthy of your time, effort, and attention.

WHAT IS THE "CARPAL TUNNEL"?

The word "carpal" refers to the wrist. Your wrist is the narrowest point on your whole arm—especially if you are a small and dainty person, but even if you are a well-built football player. The palm of the hand is much wider than the wrist is, and above it the arm gets gradually wider.

All the tendons of the arm must pass through this narrow wrist area to reach the hand. They are crowded together in a small space—the *carpal tunnel*. To protect the tendons, lubricating tissue surrounds them to minimize friction. If the tendons become inflamed by constant extension of the wrists—such as typing at a computer keyboard without wrist support—pain results. This is *carpal tunnel syndrome*.

It is particularly important to prevent or eliminate this problem if you see a back bend in your future. Your wrists must not only bend at least to 90 degrees, but also support quite a bit of weight once you push up from the floor. Strategy list for healthy wrists: strengthen them; stretch them; change faulty habits to better ones; and do the MELT® Hand Treatment (see *Further Study*, p. 185).

63 the split

ENLIST YOUR MIND

Here you will almost certainly need to think calming thoughts. Your body most probably doesn't know what has hit it. It needs time to process all the sensations it is feeling, and your mind can assist by not giving in to panic. Breathe calmly. Tell your mind it's only one minute. Close your eyes for a couple of slow breaths. The time will pass, and you will be safely on your way out of the pose.

Although working on your split is not precisely painful, the sensory stimulation takes a bit of getting used to. You can accustom your mind to this discipline—you may end up looking forward to it.

You need some upper-body strength in the beginning stages when you push on the chairs or blocks. Make sure you push with enough gentle force that you do not sink into your shoulders. Keep your shoulders dropped and your chest lifted. Relax your neck and look straight in front of you.

- **The Preparation:** Before you attempt your first split, here are the muscle groups to stretch:
  a Hamstrings: stretches 51–53.
  b Hip Flexors: stretches 35–37.
  c Quadriceps: stretches 49–50.

  Think of how a person looks sitting in a split. One leg is forward, and one leg is back. In the forward leg the hamstring muscle group is stretching; in the back leg the quadriceps and hip-flexor groups.

- **The Setup:** Prepare your stretching area. Use a floor surface with enough padding that your heel (front leg) and your knee (back leg) will not protest and distract you. You will need all your concentration when you start feeling the stretch. It is also helpful if your front heel is able to slide on the floor, mat, or carpet surface. As you sink progressively toward the floor, it is your front heel that will be making the forward adjustment.

  Line up your torso between two chairs—the folding variety is a good size. Or, if you have them, a yoga block on each side of your torso works just as well. But these are not necessary—most people will have two chairs in their home.

  Place your body in a kneeling lunge position (stretch 37), with your left leg forward and right leg back. Place your forearms on your two supporting chairs. Make sure that your forearms are comfortable: bring the chairs close to your torso so your weight will pass straight down from your shoulders into your elbows—not away from your body at an angle, because that will stress your shoulders.

  It's a good idea to have a clock or watch in view with a second hand. When you first start practicing, holding the stretch for a minute on each side is probably long enough. A mirror is also helpful, so you can check on the position of your torso during the stretch.

- **The Stretch:** When you're ready to start, take a deep breath, expanding your ribs. As you exhale, straighten your left leg and let it slide slowly forward. Adjust your chairs so they remain at a convenient distance to support your forearms.

  Keep your back upright: do *not* let it lean forward. Many people think they're doing a "split," but they are unable to sit straight up. From the very beginning of your practice—even if you are 20 in (50 cm) off the ground—be sure to keep your back tall.

Another thing you *must* do is keep your right leg (back leg) parallel. The inside of your knee will want to turn towards the floor. Do your best to keep your knee in line with your hip, and your foot in line with your knee. If you allow your knee to rotate outward, you may get more of a split sooner, but you open yourself up to knee injury. Slow and steady practice with correct alignment—both legs parallel—makes for a safer technique.

The stretch will appear, rather vehemently, in your left hamstrings and your right quadriceps and hip flexors. Keep your torso weighted between your legs—evenly over the right and left legs. Because of the intensity of this stretch, it will be immediately apparent to you whether you need more stretch in the left leg (hamstrings) or right leg (quadriceps and hip flexors).

Breathe slowly and deeply for the time allotted.

To come out of the split, do whichever of these feels more comfortable:

a   Push up with your forearms on the chair seats until you are back in your kneeling lunge.

b   Sit down gently on the floor with the left side of your butt, while your right knee bends to come out of the position.

As your level of flexibility increases, (b) will be easier than (a). Repeat the stretch on the other side.

- **Enhance Your Flexibility:** There are several techniques you can employ while you hold your split. Here are two:

a   Rotate your left (front) foot out and in. Even make little circles with your ankle. Get your body used to every angle of stretch your front leg has.

b   Do small lower-leg lifts with your right (back) foot, that is, your knee remains on the ground while you lift your foot up a little. A set of eight lifts, taking your time to feel the muscles working, and then rest.

These seem like small things, but you may be surprised at how much effort it takes to lift your back foot off the ground. The first time you try it, you may have the experience of giving your body a command that it doesn't know how to execute. This is okay. Your body is learning along with your mind, and will understand if you give it the necessary time.

Two other tips to enhance your split practice:

a   Consider starting with your less flexible side. Usually the first thing we practice gets our best attention. If you have identified that right leg forward is harder for you than left leg forward, start with the right. You will have a better chance of evening out the sides.

b   As you gradually get lower and lower over time, you will need more lower-back extension on the right (back) side. Think about what happens in the body. Your left (front) leg is already straight from the beginning, but the right (back) leg is bent. It will not completely straighten until you have enough hip-flexor range to allow total contact of the quadriceps with the floor. As the hip is able to open more and more, and the thigh sinks behind you, the curve in your sacrum/lower back gets more extreme. You will feel this happening as you progress, and it is a good idea to warm up and condition your lower-back/sacrum area in extension (stretches 15–17).

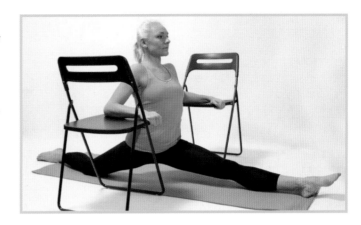

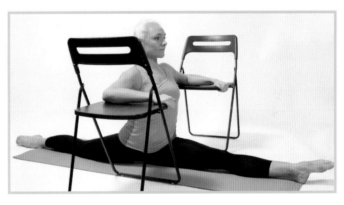

KEY
Tensor fascia lata
Rectus femoris
Semimembranosus
Semitendinosus

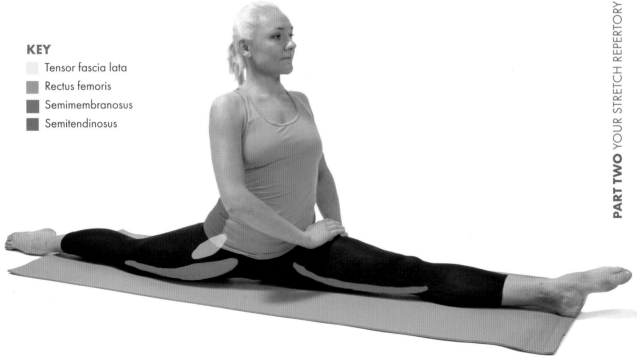

64 the back bend

ENLIST YOUR MIND

When you turn your body upside down, the world looks different. Your mind has a re-orientation job to do here. When you stand up after practicing the back bend the first few times, you may feel dizzy or have a slight headache. These will pass. Just have a chat with your mind and don't panic.

The main thing is reassuring your mind that such an unusual technique is possible for you to do. If you break it down into steps and practice consistently, a back bend is not only possible—but inevitable.

- **The Preparation:** When you prepare to practice your back bend, here are the muscle groups to stretch:
  a   Lower-back Extension: stretches 15–17.
  b   Upper-back Extension: stretches 20–21.
  c   Front Shoulder: stretches 6–7.
  d   Full-spine Extension (Sphinx): stretch 22.
  e   Wrist Extension: stretch 31.

  From the moment you push up into your first back bend, you will understand how all these muscle groups are involved. If you have a back bend in mind as a long-term goal, practice the above stretches before you undertake the back bend, until you feel your body becoming more limber in these areas.

- **The Setup:** Lie on your back on a surface that is supportive, but has enough padding to make you comfortable. Bend your knees and put your feet on the floor close to your butt. Place your palms flat on the floor by your shoulders. Heels of the hands are behind fingertips, which point toward the toes. (Immediately your wrists are in extension.)

- **The Stretch:** Take a deep breath. On the exhale, push your feet and hands into the floor and lift your body up as high as you can. Push with your feet; push with your hands; lift your hips up high. Hold for a count of eight. To come down, lower the top of your head to touch the floor and immediately tuck your chin. The back of your neck will roll gently down onto the floor. Keep pushing the floor with your hands as you lower your head, so your neck will not be taking any weight.

  The back bend is not only a triumph of flexibility, but a feat of great strength. When you first attempt to lift your body up into this extension curve, you will realize how much strength you need in your upper body to bring it off. Your legs are relatively much stronger—after all, they carry you around all the time.

  After you rest, try your back bend again; hold for a count of eight; rest. Three times in a session is plenty, until you get used to doing it.

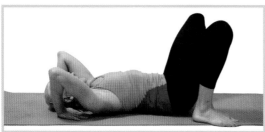

Each time you release your back bend and return to the floor, pull your knees to your chest and stretch your back the other way (in flexion). Rest between attempts; drink water; breathe.

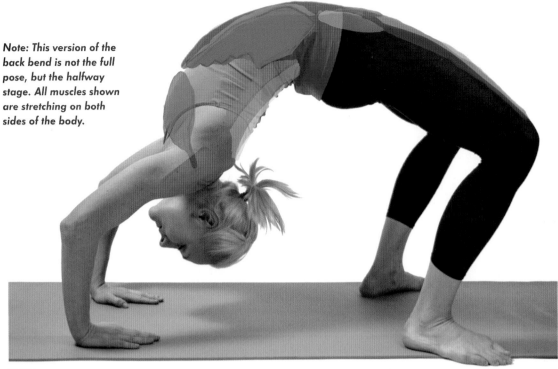

Note: This version of the back bend is not the full pose, but the halfway stage. All muscles shown are stretching on both sides of the body.

KEY

Anterior deltoid
Pectoralis major
Rectus abdominis
External oblique

Erector spinae:
Iliocostalis
Longissimus thoracis
Spinalis thoracis

Tensor fascia
lataRectus femoris

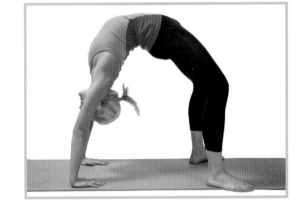

- **Enhance Your Flexibility:** Here are a couple of techniques to help you attain back-bend prowess:
  a As you gain strength in and familiarity with the position, practice shifting your weight a bit: slowly toward your feet, slowly toward your hands. This prepares you for eventual "walking" in the back bend. Do eight shifts—four each way—and then come down and rest.
  b As you increase your ability to straighten your arms (shoulder flexibility), you will be able to straighten your legs more as well, and your hip flexors will need more stretch-ability. Add the hip-flexor stretches if you feel you need them (stretches 35–37).

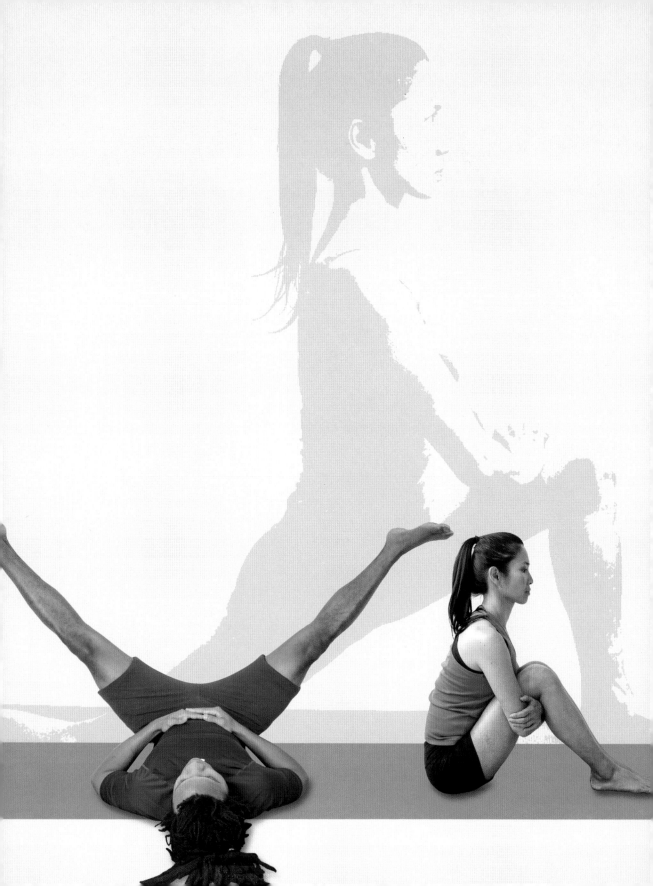

PART THREE
STRETCH SEQUENCES

Discover recipes to make with your *Part Two* ingredient mix.
Here you will find out why pursuing flexibility is a worthwhile
addition to a life that feels good while you're living it.
Do you have a particular passion for running or racquetball?
Do you experience knee pain on a regular basis? Do you
wake up stiff in the mornings? Are you determined to
get a split—or bust? And just what is a warm-up
anyway? As you dispel confusion and put together the
suggestions in these articles with your chosen *Part Two*
stretches, the mist of incomprehension around
flexibility will start to clear.

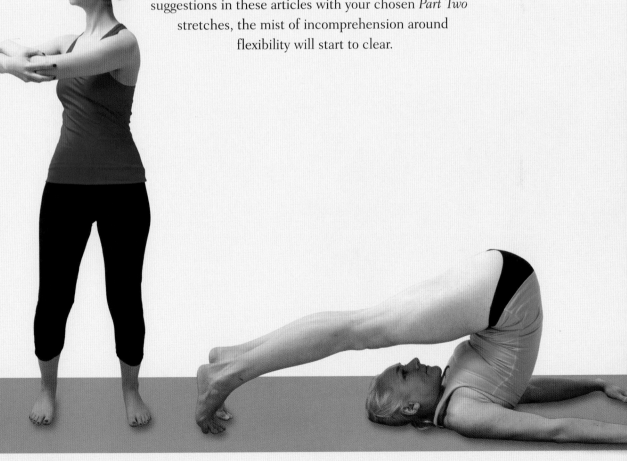

Prepare to Stretch: moving warm-ups

What is a warm-up—and why do it?

The stand-alone flexibility training session is a "real" workout—although of a different kind. Therefore, warming up will help you to get the best results from a stretching session. The increase in core and muscle temperature provided by a warm-up makes stretching safer and more productive.

It is helpful to incorporate a series of stretches into your warm-up before a physical activity—like running, for example. But stretching is not a complete warm-up—it is a warm-up component.

Just in case you are now confused, let's talk about what "warming up" before physical activity means. What should it accomplish? How does it justify the extra time it requires?

You warm up for two reasons: to prevent injury, and to prepare your body for optimum performance of a physical activity.

The warm-up accomplishes those goals by delivering the following benefits:

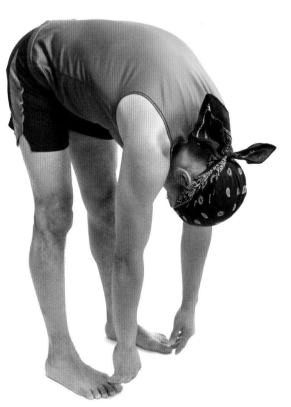

Group A

- Increases heart and respiratory rates, preparing your cardiovascular system for activity.
- Increases blood flow through your active muscles, and hence delivery of oxygen and nutrients.
- Increases nerve impulse speed, making it easier to move your body.
- Allows muscles to contract and relax faster and more efficiently.

Group B

- Increases core and muscle temperature.
- Decreases resistance to muscle stretch-ability.
- Decreases muscle tension.
- Enhances connective tissue and muscular stretch-ability.

All the above benefits assist your body to work better, but Group A is especially helpful when you are proceeding from warm-up to sports activity, and Group B when you are focusing on increasing your range of motion through stretching.

So, what exactly do you do to warm up?

Well, there are many opinions about it, but here are some guidelines:

- **First, if your chosen activity is a flexibility session,** doing five to ten minutes of some moderate-paced, general body movements will be enough to increase your body temperature. Getting warm enough to sweat is good—but getting tired during the warm-up is not. This is enough activity to prepare you for a productive stretching session—and that's what you get in this section.

- **Second, if your workout goal for the session is a more aerobically demanding physical activity**—such as running, cycling, etc.—stretch the muscle groups you will be targeting in your activity. You can accomplish this in about ten minutes (see *Stretch Before and After Common Physical Activities,* p. 142, for the muscle groups that different activities use, and for stretch duration suggestions).

- **Third, if you are on a team or practicing for an individual sporting event beyond the casual,** you may be doing some sport-specific drills as well, and finishing it all up with more stretching of the dynamic variety.

Some sports stretching experts advocate warming up for as much as 35 to 40 minutes before engaging in a sports activity. Obviously, if your entire workout time is 45 minutes or an hour, you will do a shorter warm-up.

The classic aerobic dance class always begins with an ideal warm-up:

1 Five minutes of big body movements, followed by

2 Five minutes of stretches in motion.

The beauty of (2) is that you are stretching, but you never stop moving. The warm-up prepares your body for the goal—non-stop movement for at least 45 minutes (exclusive of cool-down and ending stretch)—by warming up the core body temperature in (1) and by incorporating the appropriate stretches in (2). Perfect.

The upshot is: do you feel warm and ready to work? Dancers always say that their muscles work better in a warm room—that is, when your body and muscles feel warm, you're ready to go.

1 back

The two movements below—Spinal Roll-Down and Spinal Roll-Up—
are meant to be performed one after the other without a pause.
In a class with an instructor guiding you, this would become obvious.
But in a book, you necessarily have to read about the movements in
sequence. Read the directions first, and then execute both
movements smoothly.

As you get used to the movements, you can execute them a little
faster. Instead of counting "eight" on the way down and on the way
up, try counting a slow "four," letting your spine ripple as it moves.

1a spinal roll-down

- **The Setup:** Stand comfortably, with your feet as wide as your
  shoulders (not too narrow), your knees slightly bent, and your
  shoulders relaxed. Breathe easily and calmly.

- **The Movement:** Tuck your chin to your chest, and begin rolling
  your spine slowly down from the top of your head. Allow your extended
  arms to dangle freely, and your relaxed fingers to descend toward the floor.
  Feel each part of your body roll down in its turn. See if you can feel each
  separate bone in your back curving downward after the one above it.

    When your head passes your waistline on its way down toward the floor,
  pull your belly button in toward your spine to protect the vertebrae of your
  lower back. Keep the back of your neck extended and relaxed. Your view
  should be your legs and feet—not what's in front of you.

    Take a full eight slow counts to roll down. Stop your roll when you reach
  your maximum downward range.

    Perform three to five repetitions of the complete (a) Roll-Down and (b) Roll-
  Up sequence. Stop when you feel your spine start to become free and loose.

- **Enhance Your Experience:** You may want to start the downward movement
  using a big, exhaling sigh as you tuck your chin.

1b spinal roll-up

- **The Setup:** Perform this movement immediately after the Spinal Roll-Down.
  You will be standing with your spine bent as far down toward the floor as
  you can at this moment—without forcing. Your feet are as wide as your
  shoulders, your knees bent, your neck relaxed, your arms dangling.

ENLIST YOUR MIND

Spare half a thought for your
knees: keep them generously
bent. When we concentrate on
a principal movement—such
as rolling down the spinal
vertebrae in sequence—we
sometimes forget to check on
what the rest of our body is
doing. Bent knees: put this
signal in the back of your mind.
Thinking this helps to develop
global body awareness.

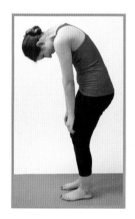

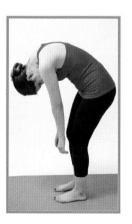

ENLIST YOUR MIND

The point of this movement is smooth, fluid execution. Make it as flowing and non-stop as you can. Lots of space between the vertebrae as you gradually become upright again. *And*—bend your knees!

- **The Movement:** Give your body the signal to roll up by pushing down into the floor slightly with your heels. At the same time, pull your belly button in to protect your spinal vertebrae as you curl them slowly up, one after the other. Your view is that of your legs and feet. Make sure not to look up—you will certainly crick your neck.

  Take a full eight slow counts to roll up. Feel your shoulders resettle themselves on your ribcage. The last thing to come up will be the top of your head.

  Perform three to five repetitions of the complete (a) Roll-Down and (b) Roll-Up sequence. Stop when you feel your spine start to become free and loose.

- **Enhance Your Experience:** As you give the impulse through your heels to start rolling up, you may want to utilize an exhaling breath. As you roll up, cultivate feeling each bone in your spine as it regains its place on top of the one below it.

2 shoulders: arm circles

- **The Setup:** Stand comfortably, with your feet as wide as your shoulders (not too narrow), your knees slightly bent, and your shoulders relaxed. Breathe easily and calmly.

- **The Movement:** Swing one arm in a great arc, first forward, then up, then back, and around to your starting place again. Use momentum: as you begin your circle, it helps to bend your knees. Use the impulse you get from straightening them slightly to swing your hand at the end of your arm.

  The idea is to move only your shoulder—your wrist and elbow joints are relaxed, your fingers loose.

  Perform a set of eight circles front to back, then a set of eight circles back to front. Repeat with the other arm. When your shoulders start to feel loose, free, and warm, you are ready to go on to the next movement.

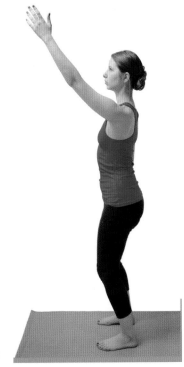

ENLIST YOUR MIND

Keep your neck relaxed and your shoulders low as you perform this movement. When you move, you always want to release unwanted tension—not create more of it.

- **Enhance Your Experience:** To help you feel the essence of this movement, think of the great circle one end of a rope makes, as you hold the other end anchored in your hand and swing it from there. Your hand is the free end of the rope. The impulse for the circle originates at the shoulder end of the movement. Your arm is dead weight—just like the other end of the rope.

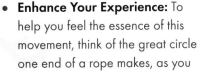

3 abdominals: side-to-side "washing machine"

- **The Setup:** Stand comfortably, with your feet as wide as your shoulders (not too narrow), your knees slightly bent, and your shoulders relaxed. Breathe easily and calmly. Extend your elbows out in front of you, with each hand grasping the opposite elbow. Keep your elbows slightly lower than shoulder height, to avoid tensing up your shoulders. You are creating a firm upper-body structure, similar to what ballroom dancers do when they connect their upper bodies to form a stable "frame."

- **The Movement:** Keeping your hips facing straight ahead, turn the rest of your upper body—from the waist upward—first to one side, then to the other. Make this a continuous movement—side to side, side to side, with your whole upper body turning at once and your hips stable.

    The idea is to feel your abdominal muscles powering the turn for you. Everything else is stable and solid—upper and lower body both—and your abs are churning right and left, like a top-loading washing machine.

    To begin, perform two set of eight repetitions (right and left is one repetition) at a fairly slow tempo. Then speed up slightly for two more sets, and slightly more again for the last two sets. This movement aims to get your core temperature up by engaging your abdominal muscles, and to access your deeper breathing.

- **Enhance Your Experience:** Turn your head in the same direction you turn your arms, looking over the midpoint of your forearms as you move. Focus to left or right as you turn to that side—this will keep you from getting dizzy.

ENLIST YOUR MIND

Hips do not move. Knees stay bent. Shoulders stay down and relaxed.

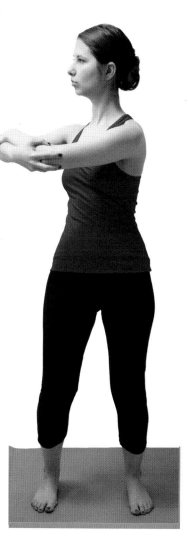

4 hips: side-to-side alternating open-knee rock, seated

- **The Setup:** Sit comfortably on the floor, with your knees wide open and your feet wider than your knees. Place your hands behind you for support and balance, and lean back until you find the best placement for your body. Just make sure that your chest remains lifted, and you do not strain your shoulders by sinking your chest between them.

- **The Movement:** Keeping one knee open, rock the other knee inward. Move the first knee outward as you rock the opposite knee inward. Take turns with your knees for a slow, continuous movement. One opens; one closes.

    Moving fairly slowly from side to side, perform two sets of eight (one repetition is left plus right). As you get to know your body better, you may decide you need two additional sets to get a sense of release and freedom in your hip joints. The number of repetitions is flexible.

- **Enhance Your Experience:** This is a hip-opening movement. Concentrate on the feeling in your hips—not on the knee movement. You do not have to drop your knee all the way to the floor. Focus instead on what's happening in your hip joint—even push your hip a little forward as you move your knee out and in. You will feel sensation toward the front and inside of your hip—not so much toward the outside or back.

    If you are not used to moving this area, you may compare the feeling in your hips to the resistance that a long-immobile rusty screw gives you when you try to unscrew it. Your hips may feel odd, and "creak" a little as they begin to loosen. Be gentle with them.

Now you're warm and ready to stretch.

ENLIST YOUR MIND

This is an uncommon movement for many people. Many of our common physical activities are parallel and linear, that is, all movement takes place in the straight-ahead, frontal plane. Think of cycling, running, etc. Give yourself time to accustom your body to the feeling of opening your hips in this side-to-side way.

prepare to stretch: moving warm-ups

141

PART THREE STRETCH SEQUENCES

Stretch before and after common physical activities

When you use stretching to help you prepare to engage in—and recover from—your favorite physical activity, it is a good idea to have a plan for what to do and how to do it. Your plan will develop as you let the various suggestions in this book roll around in your head. As ideas occur to you for applying the art of stretching to your life, you might want to make a few notes. From those notes will come your organized stretching plan.

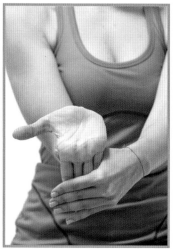

Stretch *before* the activity

As discussed in *Moving Warm-Ups* (see p. 136), stretching is an important part of warming up—but not the whole warm-up. You will be coming to stretching after five to ten minutes of moderate-paced, general body movements.

How do you decide which muscle groups to stretch?

Stretch the principal muscles used in your chosen activity. For one-side-only activities (like golf, in which your swing is usually consistently from the same side), it's a good idea to balance your body and stretch the opposite side as well. In this section we will cover a selection of physical activities done by many people—basketball, cycling, racquetball/handball, running, swimming, walking, and yoga. You will get a road map for stretching the muscles that are most relevant to performing these activities.

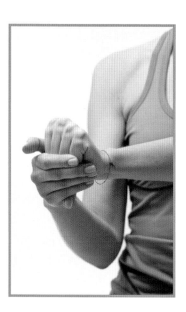

How do you stretch these muscles before their workout?

As discussed in *Part One: Ways to Stretch* (see p. 31), the goal you have in mind determines the character and duration of the stretch. For example, at this pre-workout moment, your core temperature is already raised in preparation for the physical activity to follow, so keep your body moving when you enter the stretch phase of the warm-up. Use either Shorter Static Stretching or Stretch in Motion (see *Part One: Ways to Stretch*, p. 31, for more detail).

Stretch *after* the activity

Immediately after doing an intense physical activity is a terrific time for you to increase your muscles' range of motion. As discussed in *Part One: Why Stretch?* (p. 16), this benefit of regular flexibility practice not only decreases your likelihood of injury, but increases your ability to excel at the activities you love.

Before you stretch, make sure you first cool down. If your activity has been intense, you have been living at a heightened level of reality (for example, "runner's high"). Do some moderate-paced, full-body movements to bring your body back down to its normal state. (This is similar to "hot-walking" a thoroughbred after a race—absolutely essential to the horse's muscular health. Your muscles will not be happy either if you don't cool them down gradually after an intense workout.)

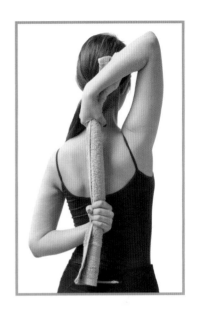

Which muscle groups do you stretch?

As stated in *Stretch Before the Activity*, opposite, identify and stretch the principal muscles used in your chosen activity. For one-side-only activities, balance your body by stretching the opposite side as well. In this section, we cover the main muscle groups important for basketball, cycling, racquetball/handball, running, swimming, walking, and yoga. Use this road map as a guide to stretching the muscles that are most relevant when you do these activities.

How do you stretch these muscles after their workout?

As discussed in *Part One: Ways to Stretch* (see p. 31), your stretching goal determines the type and duration of the stretch. Here, in the post-workout situation, your core temperature is starting to drop and your muscles are cooling down. Your body is returning to equilibrium, its natural state. Some research indicates that, if you can keep your muscles in an elongated position while they are cooling down, they will be more likely to retain their newly lengthened status permanently. Explore how the following methods work for you: Longer Static Stretching, PNF Stretching, or Rhythmic Breathing (see *Part One: Ways to Stretch*, p. 31, for more detail).

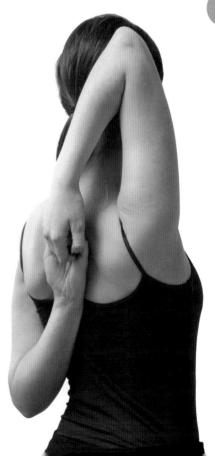

Use stretch to improve your activity performance

There is a wealth of information available on each topic covered here. Sifting through it is a huge undertaking. Even among experts in the field, the same person may disagree with himself in two different articles. Entire books exist to guide you through each activity as you become a competent exerciser or player. And of course, to be really prepared for movement, we should stretch practically every muscle in the body, since most of them are used in every sport in an integrated way.

In the limited space available here, we will focus on one or two skills necessary to execute each activity safely and well. The suggested stretches in each section are aimed at helping you to improve only the specifically mentioned aspects of playing your sport or doing your favorite activity.

Often, the skills needed for one activity transfer well to another, so you can get more mileage out of the suggestions offered here. For example, the ability to dart quickly and stop on a dime, discussed in the section on racquetball/handball, is equally valuable when applied to basketball.

Muscles used in most activities

To keep you from being overwhelmed as you start a stretching practice, the recommended stretches in each activity section usually do not exceed five main and three bonus ones. The following muscles are important for almost every activity. They may have been left out of the list for a particular activity (usually because other stretches need addressing first) but, if you want to expand the number of stretches you do, consider these.

Buttocks

Stretching these muscles is universally important because they:

- Help maintain the correct lumbar curve. They pull on the lower back when tight, causing that lumbar curve to flatten. Those spinal discs become more vulnerable to compression by the upright spine. This is compounded for athletes who perform extraordinary movements.

- Help rotate the hips easily. Although golf is the obvious example here, you can make the case that all our listed activities use hip rotation extensively. (Even swimming, which uses hip rotation to increase hand force against the water.)

Feet

Stretching the feet improves the range of movement in the foot and calf for cardiovascular activity (any sport, basically).

Here is our short list of common physical activities and the muscle groups most relevant to doing them well.

Basketball

A good basketball player is able to move effortlessly in any direction at any moment. Play changes course constantly, and the player must be able to adjust quickly. Freedom of movement of the spine and hips allows the player to develop this skill.

Another essential component of the basketball skill package is mastering the all-important jump.

Here is a set of stretches to help you gain the flexibility you need to go after these two skills of the game (as well as some bonus skills helped by the same stretches).

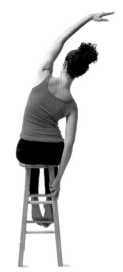

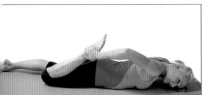

1 back: spiral, stretch 24c
skills improved: changing direction, driving to basket

2 back: side, stretch 23
skills improved: changing direction, driving to basket

Bonus stretches

Also try these for improving your jump. And, of course, add or substitute any stretches you feel work better for you.

1 abdominals: torso lift from floor, stretch 26
skills improved: jump

2 calves: leg straight, stretch 55a
skills improved: jump

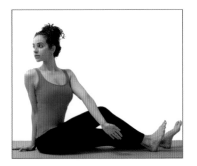

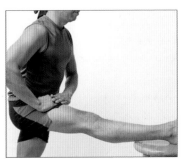

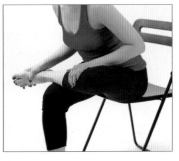

3 thighs: quadriceps, stretch 49
skills improved: changing direction, jump, sprinting

4 thighs: hamstrings, stretch 53
skills improved: changing direction, jump, sprinting

5 hips: buttocks, stretch 38
skills improved: jump

Cycling

Your ability to move smoothly through the two phases of the pedal stroke—propulsion and recovery—is a major skill you develop in cycling. You must get your muscle groups to move continuously, as long as your bicycle is in motion, with the least deviation from the ideal position for your body. To maintain the seamless flow of this motion, several muscle groups are involved—and they work on every stroke of the pedal.

When muscles work non-stop against a load—as happens in cycling, especially going up hills—they automatically gain in strength. In cycling, your muscles never get a chance to extend fully. Even when your foot is as close to the ground as the stroke allows, your knee is still

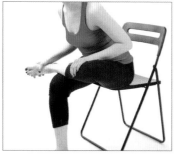

1 hips: buttocks, stretch 38
muscle role: especially when you stand in the saddle

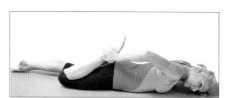

2 thighs: quadriceps, stretch 49
muscle role: especially going up hills

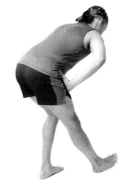

3 thighs: hamstrings, stretch 51
muscle role: work with quadriceps to power pedaling

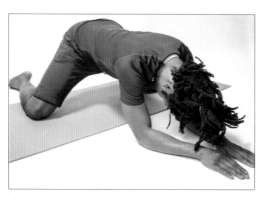

4 inner thighs, stretch 46
muscle role: hold your knees in line with your feet and hips for a more efficient pedal cycle

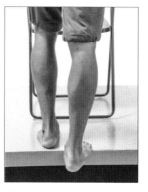

5 calves: leg straight, stretch 55a
calves: knee bent, stretch 55b
muscle role: both upper and lower—assist in pedaling

slightly bent. To prevent your working muscles from getting tighter and tighter, and ending up by inhibiting the ease of your stroke execution, call these stretching techniques into play.

Stretching can enhance your overall ability to cycle well. When you lengthen muscles systematically—a little beyond the absolute range they need to perform the activity—their increased range of motion does away with any resistance that would occur with stiffer muscles. Therefore, your stroke becomes smoother and goes like clockwork.

Try putting the stretches in this section into your regular pre- and post-cycling routine, and compare how you feel once you have done it a few times with how your muscles felt before. Be alert to discovering other stretches to add or substitute that will work even better for you than the ones on this list.

Bonus stretches

Here are some other muscle groups and the function they perform when you cycle:

1 shoulders: front, stretch 7
muscle role: held in a constant position—always slightly "rounded." This stretch will open them up.

2 abdominals: torso lift from floor, stretch 26
muscle role: keep your back straight and balanced. Their stability lends power to your turns and lets you control the bike from a still and solid center.

3 hip flexors: kneeling lunge, stretch 37
muscle role: assist the quadriceps to pull your knee up before each downstroke. Can become very sore from the constant work.

Racquetball and handball

For these sports (and for tennis, for the most part), check the chart below to see the movement patterns they use and what muscles support those patterns. If the muscle group is not mentioned in the text below, and you feel the need to stretch that area, refer to the appropriate section in the *Contents* on pp. 4–6 for stretches to use.

MOVEMENT PATTERNS

PATTERN	MOBILE HIPS*	HAMSTRINGS	BUTTOCKS	LOWER BACK	CORE (ROTATIONAL ABILITY)
Backpedaling	X	X	X	X	
Cutting	X				
Darting and stopping suddenly	X				
Sprinting		X			
Swinging	X				X

*"Mobile hips" includes: hip flexors, hamstrings, buttocks, inner thighs, quadriceps, side hips.

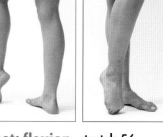

1 back: spiral, stretch 24b
muscle role: improves the ability to rotate torso for an easy, fluid swing

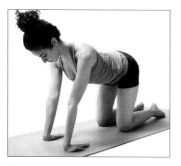

2 wrists: extension,
stretch 31
muscle role: releases the wrist from its locked position on the racquet (in handball, the wrist tendons may take a beating)

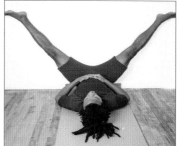

3 inner thighs, stretch 48
muscle role: enable fluid side-to-side movements

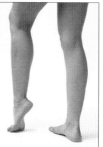

4 feet: flexion, stretch 56
feet: extension, stretch 57
muscle role: allow sudden stopping and starting

Handball special note: Stretch your hands for this sport. Your hand is your racquet. Stretches 33 and 34 are the ticket.

Tennis special note: Since the tennis court is much bigger than either the racquetball or handball court, the muscles that enable the backpedaling pattern work much harder. If you play tennis, you can probably benefit from some extra attention to:

- Hamstrings—stretches 51–53
- Buttocks—stretches 38–40
- Lower-back flexion—stretches 11–14

Bonus stretches

Here are some other muscle groups and the function they perform during racquet sports and handball:

1 upper back: flexion, stretch 18
muscle role: aids a powerful swing in the serving arm (especially in handball)

2 side hip: seated, stretch 43
muscle role: active in constant, darting movements (especially in tennis)

3 hip flexors: kneeling lunge,
stretch 37
muscle role: enable quick response from buttocks, hamstrings, and lower back when moving in multiple directions

Running

This is a straight-ahead, forward-moving activity—except perhaps for the occasional pothole or nature obstacle to duck. It has none of the side-to-side darting movements of the court sports. For most enjoyment in running, you want to cultivate the most rapid turnover of which your legs are capable—cover the most distance in the shortest time. You get better at this when you stretch your back and hips.

Whether you are sprinting, particularly care about winning your race, or are just running

for the fun of the thing, your stride will feel most comfortable when the range of motion it requires is well within your capability. You will have less muscular resistance to contend with if your muscles are used to moving beyond the minimum range necessary for your activity.

Hence, your gait becomes fluid and easy; you move with efficiency and confidence.

What the lower body does

The running stride has three phases: support, drive, and recovery.

During the *support* phase, the heel is set down on the ground, followed by the rest of the foot. There is a moment when the whole foot is flat on the ground.

Next is the *drive* phase, when the heel comes up and the ball of the foot pushes off the ground—engaging the upper and lower calves.

In the *recovery* phase, the foot is suspended above the ground. The hip flexors contract to lift the foot off the ground in the first half.

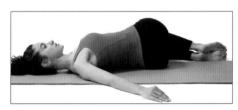

1 back: spiral, stretch 24a

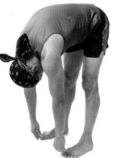

2 side hip: lying on side, stretch 42

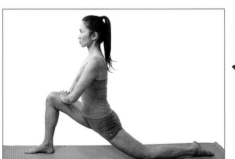

3 hip flexors: kneeling lunge, stretch 37

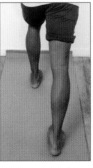

4 thighs: hamstrings, stretch 52

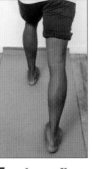

5 calves: floor, leg straight, stretch 54a
calves: support, knee bent, stretch 55b

In the last half of recovery, the hamstrings and buttocks stretch as the leg extends and the foot reaches towards the ground—and then they contract as the heel sets down again.

The upper body's role

The stars of the running show are the muscles of the lower body. Your upper body has a supporting role. It maintains your balance and keeps propelling you forward. When you run faster, your arm and shoulder opposite to the working leg gently come forward as a counterbalance. The spine gently rotates compactly from side to side.

Bonus stretches

Also experiment with the stretches below to improve your running performance ease. Add or substitute any stretches you feel are working better for you.

1 upper back: flexion, stretch 19

2 lower back: flexion, stretch 14

3 thighs: quadriceps, stretch 49

Swimming

The shoulder complex is used heavily in swimming. It is an inherently unstable structure. When our body in its wisdom designed this marvelous mechanism, it chose mobility over stability—the shoulder joint is extremely mobile, but is dependent for its stability on dynamic stabilization (muscles) and static stabilization (cartilage, ligaments, and capsules). When you prepare for a swimming workout or competition, you must be careful not to destabilize the shoulder complex right before you work it, or you could induce shoulder pain.

Avoid:

- Stretches that actually stretch the joint capsule (stretches 7–9 in this book).

- Stretching methods that don't really warm up the area—such as static stretching.

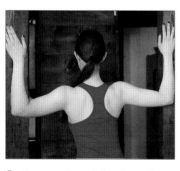

1 chest: shoulder level, stretch 10a

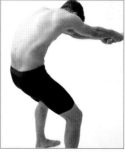

2 upper back: flexion, stretch 19

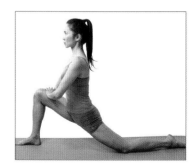

3 hip flexors: kneeling lunge, stretch 37

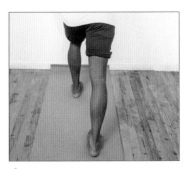

4 calves: floor, leg straight, stretch 54a

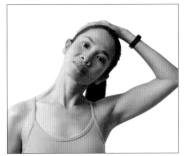

5 neck: side, stretch 1

Bonus stretch

Also experiment with the stretch below to give your neck some relief from constantly turning to the same side in the crawl stroke.

neck: back diagonal, stretch 3

Do instead:

- Stretches that target the muscles of the shoulder complex (like stretches 1 and 2 in this sequence).
- Stretching methods designed to prime your muscles to work—such as stretch in motion (or dynamic stretching, also called "mobility drills" in sport).

So, the swimming warm-up is a special case. Although the moving warm-ups in this book are fine as preparation for most physical activities (see *Moving Warm-Ups*, p. 136), they are general in nature and should be supplemented by moving warm-ups tailored for the activity of swimming.

Specific moving shoulder warm-ups for swimming[1]

- Rotator cuff (two techniques).
- Pull shoulder blades together in back.
- Pull elbows together in center and open.
- Shoulder press with overhead streamline.

Timing of stretching[2]

Separate sustained stretching from workouts and competition—such as:

- Several hours before your swimming workout.
- Several hours after your practice.
- When your muscles are not fatigued after a serious workout—such as on a cross-training or lighter swimming day.

When you consider choices about how to make stretching part of your workout, there is no substitute for your own research, which includes advice from advanced athletes and/or coaches. Gather your data; consider all angles—and make your decision.

Because—even the experts disagree with each other. One opinion (stated above) is to wait several hours after your practice before you do static stretching. Another is: do static stretching during your post-workout cool-down period, to help muscles recover immediately and decrease the likelihood of injury. To wrap up:

- Prepare for a vigorous workout—use dynamic stretching to prime your muscles and move more efficiently.
- Relax, let the muscles recover after a workout —use static stretching to improve your long-term performance.

Finally, pay attention to your hip flexors, which can become tight because of all the flutter kicking swimmers do.

Walking

Presumably, everyone knows how to walk. If walking is your exercise, however, you need muscular endurance, so you can keep moving and get aerobic benefit. Walking is the quintessential repetitive-motion activity par excellence. You need balance—which sounds negligible until you try to negotiate a steady pace on uneven terrain. You will balance better if your lower legs are strong and flexible. Remember, muscle flexibility increases muscle strength: a stretched muscle encounters less resistance as it moves through the range of motion that an activity requires.

Race walking is an intense and disciplined form of walking—heightened to the nth degree. Any muscular soreness you encounter in walking for health probably magnifies when you race-walk. Therefore, let's take this example as a good indication of which muscles to stretch— and why they may be sore from this activity.

- **Shins (anterior calves)** When you practice the proper technique for race walking, your shins will likely inform you that they have been doing something unusual. Try this at home: extend your leg forward and land on your heel

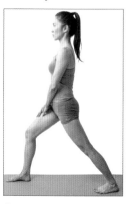

1 thighs: hamstrings, stretch 53
importance: high
intensity: low

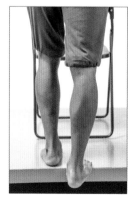

2 thighs: quadriceps, stretch 49
importance: high
intensity: medium

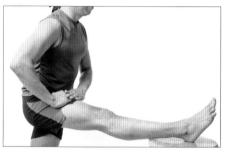

3 hip flexors: standing lunge, stretch 36
importance: high
intensity: low

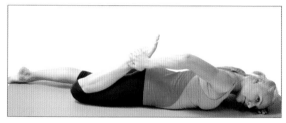

4 calves: leg straight, stretch 55a
importance: high
intensity: low

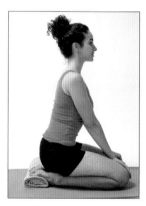

5 ankles: extension stretch 58
importance: medium
intensity: medium

with your ankle flexed. Then roll smoothly through your foot—still holding your toes up in the ankle flex. Your front calf muscles do not relax until your whole foot is on the ground. Imagine repeating this over and over, multiplied by as many strides as you take. This is clearly training of a different sort. Those front calf muscles are likely to experience soreness, and stretching is your friend in this situation.

- **Hamstrings** work especially to keep your gait even on variable terrain.

- **Shoulders** Race-walking technique moves the arms over a greater front-to-back distance than is even used by runners. Here we have upper-body repetitive motion that may result in some soreness, which you can remedy by stretching. Stretch 9 (back shoulder) is in the bonus stretch list right. But if you notice other areas of soreness, pull the appropriate stretch—for example, stretch 18 for upper back, or stretch 6 for front shoulder.

For the stretch sequence on the previous page, use the high-importance stretches after every workout. Do the stretches of lesser importance (a) if your muscles feel tight after your walking session; or (b) alternate them on different days to keep all the relevant muscles adequately flexible.

Intensity refers to how strong a stretch you feel in the targeted muscles. If you are new to stretching, or notice a particularly tight area, keep the intensity low. Up the intensity once you feel how much stretch your body can handle in a particular muscle group.

Race-walking trivia

Shin muscles work harder in walking than in almost any other sport. Usually, the only athletes to escape anterior calf soreness are equestrians. The heel-down-in-stirrups stance used in riding requires them to use these muscles to assist their balance in the saddle.

Further information

The importance/intensity information in this section is adapted from www.racewalk.com/Stretching/Introduction.asp and following pages.

For more complete information on race walking, visit www.racewalk.com/defaultRW.asp.

Bonus stretches

Particularly in race walking, you are using most of the lower-body musculature. Here are a few more stretches to incorporate, based on your own experience. Basically: if it's sore after you walk, stretch it (see above box for more information).

1 shoulders: back, stretch 9
importance: low
intensity: low

2 hips: buttocks, stretch 38
importance: medium
intensity: high

3 side hip: knee push, stretch 41
importance: medium
intensity: medium

Yoga

Yoga as a fitness activity has gained widespread acceptance over the years. The history of its ascendance in the West may be a fascinating area to explore. Every gym now has some form of yoga on its class schedule—and usually several types.

Warming up

Yoga is popularly perceived as a stretching activity, so the topic of what muscles to stretch before you do it has not really been addressed in any detail. There are many styles of yoga—some more or less strenuous (or more or less traditional) than others.

A partial list includes:

- **Ashtanga** Vigorous, with continuous movement—the sequence never varies: the more you do it, the more will be revealed about how to do it
- **Yoga nidra** All about the mind
- **YogaFit** Cardiovascular workout
- **Arco Yoga** Aerial yoga
- **Bhakti yoga** Divine worship
- **Kirtan** Devotional group chanting

Obviously, devotional chanting needs less body preparation than a cardiovascular workout. Your core temperature should be up and your major muscle groups prepared, so the information in *Moving Warm-Ups*, p. 136, will be helpful.

Here are a few warm-up suggestions from experienced yoga teacher Michael McArdle:

- Squats with proper alignment (10 reps).
- Shoulder circumductions (20 reps both directions) (see *Moving Warm-Ups*, p. 136).
- Pelvic neutral locating (the MELT® Method is great for this).
- Balancing on one foot and finding a good eye line for "spotting."
- Light hamstring stretching (see the stretch sequence on p. 155).

The role of flexibility

The focus in yoga is squarely on the practice, which may have a spiritual aspect. Although many people gain flexibility by doing yoga, this is more of a by-product than a goal. Many practitioners are drawn to yoga knowing its reputation for developing flexibility, but this is not the primary focus of the discipline.

During my fitness career, I have encountered a number of people who have attempted to adopt yoga as part of their fitness regimen, have gotten injured in the course of doing it, and consequently have given it up. Because yoga emphasizes putting yourself into a particular posture, your more flexible muscles may compensate for your less flexible ones—the ones unable to lengthen enough in the posture. You may look as though you are in the pose, but a knowledgeable teacher can examine your body and determine if muscular compensation is going on. If the flexibility disparity is great enough, your more limber areas may extend so far as to stretch stabilizers that shouldn't be stretched—that is, ligaments—and compromise the integrity of the body. This may account for the incidence of injury when inflexible people adopt a yoga practice to increase their flexibility level.

Another reason to do some pre- and post-yoga stretching is to loosen consistently tight areas. This will be individual. As discussed in *Part One: How Muscles Stretch* (see p. 22), not only are there flexibility differences between any two people, but in any one body, there are differences in the relative flexibility of body areas. If you notice that the side of your hip feels tight, preventing you from entering fully into a yoga pose, refer to *Part Two: Your Stretch Repertory* (see p. 42) and select the applicable stretches to address side-hip flexibility—and hence, improve your yoga pose.

Try the stretch sequence below as a rough guide. These muscles must be capable of flexing or stretching in various yoga poses.

Feel free to adapt the list—add, change, keep notes. Since there is a myriad of yoga styles, pay attention to your own experience and use it. Find the limiting muscular factor—and expand that area with stretch.

(see p. 22), (see p. 42)

Bonus stretches

Here are a couple of other suggestions for muscle groups that may feel tight during your yoga practice. Remember: add or substitute any stretches you feel are working better for you.

1 inner thighs, stretch 46

2 hip flexors: knee to chest, stretch 35

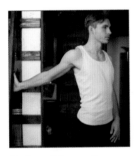

1 shoulders: front, stretch 7

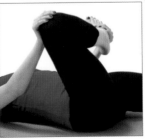

2 lower back: flexion, stretch 13

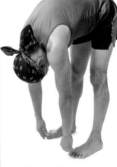

5 thighs: hamstrings, stretch 52

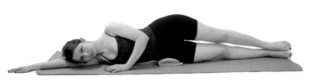

3 side hip: lying on side, stretch 42

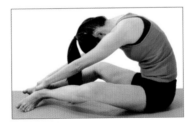

4 hips: buttocks, stretch 39

Stretch throughout your day

This section is meant to help you formulate ways stretching can improve the way your body feels as you live your day. For each sample daily activity, there is a short set of recommended stretches you can try. The sequence may work well for you as it stands. Or you may want to refer to the stretch list in *Part Two: Your Stretch Repertory* (see p. 42) to locate other stretches that may work better.

The topics discussed below are general and fairly universal (mostly everybody wakes up and goes to sleep). Use these general activities to spark some ideas of your own. How can your daily tasks benefit from the addition of stretching?

Upon waking in the morning

When you first get up in the morning, you have basically been in a static position for a number of hours. The human body tends to get stiff when it spends a long time in the same position—it would rather be moving. Take this first opportunity at the opening of your day to wake up your muscles with some gentle stretching. If you have prepared your spine adequately for sleeping (see *Before Going to Sleep*, p. 160), your spinal discs should now be uncompressed compared to the previous night. Your spine is ready to respond well to your stretching wake-up call.

The following stretches will give you a place to start as you begin to incorporate this kind of movement into the fabric of your daily life. As you become more aware of the relative flexibility or tightness of various areas of your body, you can add a few more techniques to this list, or substitute others that work better for you.

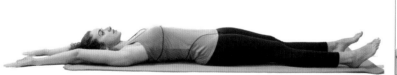

1 abdominals: finger-and-toe reach, stretch 25

2 lower back: flexion, stretch 11a

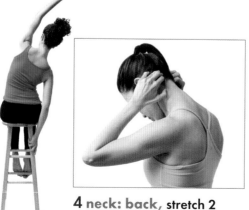

3 back: side, stretch 23

4 neck: back, stretch 2

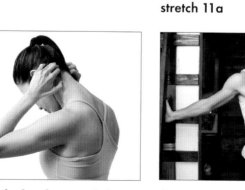

5 shoulders: front, stretch 7

Using the computer

The widespread use of the computer is a sign of our times. It is becoming by far the most efficient way of accomplishing so much in our technologically fast-paced world; indeed, many would consider it a necessity if we don't want to be left behind—either professionally or socially.

As amazing and useful as the computer is, its extensive use creates challenges for our bodies. It is easy to concentrate so completely on the screen that we lose awareness of what's happening with our body posture. We let our lower backs slump, our shoulders round, our chins jut forward to create "turtle neck." Prolonged use of the computer mouse without adequate support can wreak havoc with our wrists and hands (carpal tunnel syndrome— a repetitive-motion disorder—can be a

consequence). And of course, there is a lot of sitting involved, making our lower-back/hamstring connection inflexible. Allowing ourselves to remain in habitual postures detrimental to maintaining our optimal structure can actually change our bodies' perception of "normal." We possess a very adaptive life partner in our body, and if we stay in the "wrong" position long enough, that position begins to feel "right" to the body.

The list of stretches below will help you keep that from happening. Add whatever additional stretch techniques you discover that will help you to counteract the not-so-wonderful consequences of using the computer. Or exchange the ones following for others that work better for you.

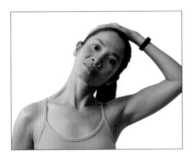

1 neck: side, stretch 1

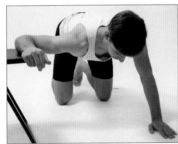

2 shoulders: front, stretch 6

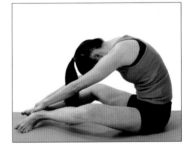

3 lower back: flexion, stretch 13

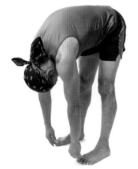

4 thighs: hamstrings, stretch 52

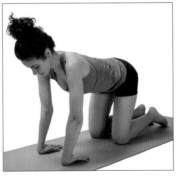

5 wrists: flexion, stretch 32

Prolonged sitting

In these times, we live in a culture of sitting. We sit for large parts of our day—in an office; on an airplane; in a car, bus, or commuter train; or watching TV. Our hunting and gathering days are behind us, but our bodies are still hardwired to move. Motion is our default mode. Most of us have experienced sitting immobile for a period of time, and then, when we signal our body to move, feeling its momentary reluctance to execute our command. Our muscles have become stiff from being held in one position too long. Sitting sessions can also cause muscular tension, an "antsy" feeling in your legs—and even pain.

When you stand up after a lengthy bout of sitting, you may automatically feel like extending your arms up toward the ceiling. This is a normal reaction: your body wants to re-lengthen itself following the curtailment of its native propensity to move.

You can build on this reaction by doing the next group of stretches. We concentrate here on the lower-back/hamstring connection, thighs, and hips. As you try other stretches in this book, and find the ones that most effectively counteract the ill effects of sitting, add them to the list below—or substitute those that work better for you.

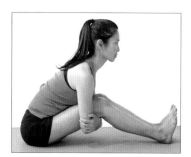

1 lower back: flexion,
stretch 14

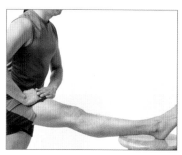

2 thighs: hamstrings,
stretch 53

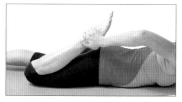

3 thighs: quadriceps,
stretch 49

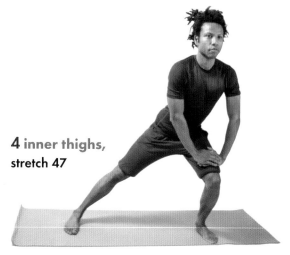

4 inner thighs,
stretch 47

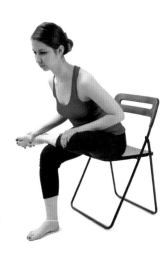

5 hips: buttocks,
stretch 38

Driving

Driving is a special subset of sitting. You can use all the stretches recommended for *Prolonged Sitting* (see opposite). But how is your sitting situation as a driver different from the passenger's? One leg is always extended forward, with your foot touching one of the pedals. Your foot hovers over the accelerator, or over the brake, or—if you drive a stick shift—it must be ready to push in the clutch pedal as well. Your hip, leg, and foot never relax. They are always ready to respond to whatever happens on the road.

This means that your legs are under unequal tension, for one thing. Your pedal leg is always extended and tense. This constant, muscles-ready-to-act state can produce a sense of strain and even soreness in your hip and/or thigh muscles.

The stretches below will help to remedy this situation. Be sure to do the stretches on both legs to lengthen them equally. As a bonus, you can also stretch your neck (stretches 1–5) and/or fingers (stretches 33–34), should you notice tightness in those areas as well. And as always, when you find techniques that work for you, include them in your session or substitute them for the ones below.

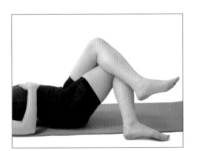

1 side hip: knee push, stretch 41

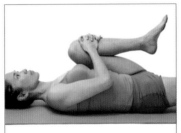

2 hip flexors: knee to chest, stretch 35

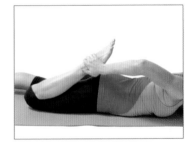

3 thighs: quadriceps, stretch 49

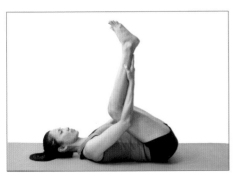

4 lower back: flexion, stretch 11b

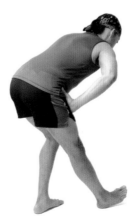

5 thighs: hamstrings, stretch 51

Before going to sleep

Sleep is of the first importance to our health. This is the daily time of repair and healing for the body. Therefore, you want to set yourself up for the optimal sleep experience, and you can use stretching as a tool to help you create just that.

After a day of living in the human upright posture, your spinal discs are necessarily compressed by your body's weight. This means you have lost precious cerebrospinal fluid from between them. This fluid is like lubricating oil between your discs, making movement effortless and light. When you sleep in the horizontal position, your spinal discs decompress, and your fluid cushion returns.

However, if the muscles around your spine are too tight, they may not be able to release enough to allow this vital fluid replenishment. You want to make this fluid exchange happen, because it is instrumental in how refreshed you feel in the morning.

So, the stretches in this section concentrate on lengthening your spine in every direction in which it can move. We want to make sure that your spine can take full advantage of the nightly healing opportunity sleep affords.

Your spine can flex (bend forward), extend (lift and bend backward), flex laterally right and left (bend sideways), and rotate right and left. Also included is your cervical spine (neck). Use the sequence below to free your spine before you sleep—and, of course, add or substitute other stretch techniques that work well for you.

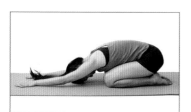

1 lower back: flexion, stretch 12

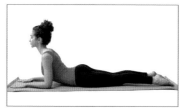

2 back: extension, stretch 22

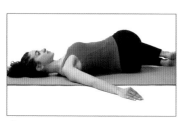

4 back: spiral, stretch 24a

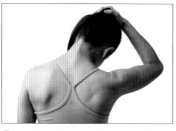

5 neck: back diagonal, stretch 3

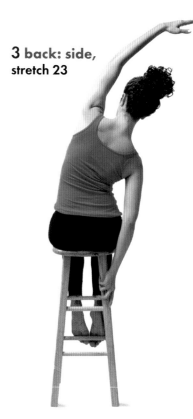

3 back: side, stretch 23

Stretch to relieve common areas of pain

In my experience, recovering from any pain is a road that every person travels individually. You can get to know your body's signals. How is this pain different from your other experiences of low-spine pain? Is it soreness from exercise overwork? Sharp pain that indicates injury? Dull, persistent pain that doesn't seem to be related to muscles at all? It is possible to tune in to your body, to develop a working partnership with it. No one else has your precise combination of body and mind. Basically, you try what you know and see what that does. Use the feedback from the techniques you've already tried when you plan your next step.

Consider this

Pain is your body's cry for help—your help. It's a signal in your body's repertoire of ways to contact you. Your body seems to be all around you, but try out an image of it as a small someone asking for help—like a child. Before a child becomes verbal in the adult way, a parent figures out what it's "saying" by watching and listening. A wordless communication system is operating. Ditto with your body. It's saying, "I'm hurting. I'll give you clues to help you figure it out."

Work with your body

Attend closely to your body. How it feels will tell you how long to hold a position. If a body part is in really acute pain, don't sweat it. Stretch *around* the painful area, adding a very gentle, experimental approach to the part that's actually painful. Working to remedy pain is different from working to increase range of motion. Go easy.

Do each stretch on both sides, even though you may feel the pain only on one side. Always cultivate balance in the body. Imbalance is a step on the road to injury.

Work with your mind

When you seek to remedy pain, use primarily gentle stretches. You are coaxing the body out of a condition of pain. Especially in a state like this, in which you are getting a clear signal from your body that it's seeking your help, remember that it is likely to respond better to low-key nudging and prodding than to force. Ask your body what it wants by feeling into the area with your mind. Do you need to shift the angle a little? Apply slightly more or less intensity? Closing your eyes might enhance your ability to feel.

Complementary healing tools

Stretching knowledge is a real ace in the hole for you. It may not be the whole answer to your particular brand of pain, so consider stocking your personal healing kit with other tools. For example:

- A gentle massage—olive oil with a few drops of a pure, relaxing aromatherapy oil mixed in, such as lavender. Non-professional massage works well here, although you can enlist the help of a massage therapist.
- A relaxing, de-stress bath, again including an agent such as Epsom salt or calming aromatherapy oils.
- Another healing modality you may be familiar with, of which there are many. Gyrokinesis® and The MELT Method® are two that work well (see p. 185 for more on both of these).

Muscular (or joint) pain has myriad causes. It can happen because of anything from a sudden accidental fall or twist to just using the muscle too intensely or for too long. Some possible causes of pain are mentioned in each section, but the list can be as long as there are situations in life.

Generally, when you consider employing the modality of stretching to remedy pain, remember that the time to bring stretching into the healing picture is after severe pain has subsided. If you have an acute injury, start treatment with R.I.C.E.—Rest, Ice, Compression, and Elevation—for 48 to 72 hours after the event.

Depending on the severity of the injury, you may elect to seek medical advice, which is likely to be: start healing the area with heat and gentle massage. But you may want to reassure yourself by consulting a specialist. You can start this next stage of treatment after 48 to 72 hours.

When you feel the acute stage passing and the pain has become much less, you can introduce stretching techniques to bring the muscles back up to their original flexibility level.

Neck and shoulder

Neck

Your neck pain may originate from habits that place extra stress on your neck, for example:

- Cocking your head to one side during a phone conversation.
- Tilting your head down when you read or text. Jutting out your chin as you work on the computer.
- Hunching up your shoulders without being aware you are doing it.

Your head is heavy, and it balances best on your body when your neck has a slight backward curve. Your neck muscles will become strained if you habitually lean your head forward.

Stretching can help relieve neck pain, but also pay attention to the ways you hold your neck. Changing from a detrimental to a beneficial neck posture will help the stretches do their work.

Try the stretches below—gently. Less intense is better than more intense. Explore the range your neck has, instead of forcing your neck into the stretch position with violent pulling.

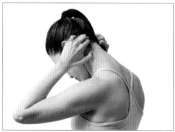
1 neck: back, stretch 2

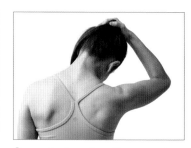
2 neck: back, diagonal, stretch 3

Shoulder

A few possible causes of shoulder pain might be:

- Neck pain that radiates down into your shoulders.
- Carrying heavy bags or suitcases. This is a workout for your trapezius muscles, but you may also be unaware that you are causing them unnecessary stress by hiking up your shoulders instead of letting them relax (this may also contribute to neck pain).
- Working out your shoulders (which stresses the area) without adequate shoulder flexibility. This may cause nagging, annoying pain that is different from post-exercise muscle soreness. The location of the pain may migrate—it may seem to move from the front to the back, for example.

The following two stretches can help with this pain. They can also help to prevent frozen shoulder (painful, stiff shoulder with possible loss of full shoulder movement range). If you are not used to stretching your shoulders, when you start it may feel as though the remedy is worse than the malady. It can be painful when you start to open a stiff area that has never been addressed before. Be very gentle with the shoulder stretches below. Massaging the shoulder with a little olive oil and a few added drops of a relaxing essential oil can also help.

Stretching methods for neck and shoulder pain:

- Rhythmic Breathing (see p. 32)
- Static Stretching (see pp. 32–33)

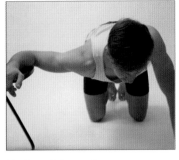

1 shoulders: front, stretch 6

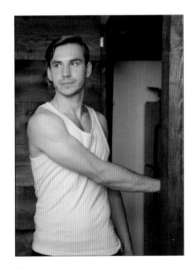

2 shoulders: back, stretch 8

Next steps

When the pain condition improves, you can add some intensity to the stretches in this neck and shoulder section. But always continue to monitor how your neck and shoulder feel, so you will be relieving pain—not causing it.

Lower back and sacrum

Pain in the spinal areas known as the lower back (around your waistline) and the sacrum (below your waistline) is very common. Pain in this area can arise from:

- A sudden muscular effort that you are not used to making (weight training helps avoid this!).
- Lack of strength in abdominal muscles.
- Shortening in the hip-flexor muscles, which may pull the low-spine muscles into a habitual angle that they are not designed to sustain.
- Weakness (or tightness) in another area of the body, for which the body is compensating by putting extra strain on the low spine, as in injury recovery, when muscles on the injured side of the body work harder while the injured side rests.
- Gut problems. Sounds unlikely, but the nerves that affect the gut "speak" through the spine. That means, if your digestion is off, the body may tell you about it with spinal soreness.
- Other stuff I didn't mention.

With so many possible causes, doing stretches may not be the whole solution. There is no magic bullet, no free lunch.

Even though that's true, a working knowledge of which stretches can potentially help is a valuable tool in your personal healing kit. In particular, pay attention to the hamstring/low-back connection, which is often a key factor when you address low-spine pain relief.

We are working around the hip before addressing the actual pain site. Often, the stress or imbalance that may be causing the pain is located somewhere distant from where you feel it.

Next steps

When the pain condition improves, you could substitute more intense stretches for some of those pictured below, e.g:

1 hip flexors: standing lunge, stretch 36

2 thighs: hamstrings, stretch 53

3 lower back: flexion, stretch 11b

4 lower back: flexion, stretch 12

Upper-back tension or imbalance may also be involved in low-spine pain. Experiment with these stretches:

1 upper back: flexion, stretch 18

2 upper back: flexion, stretch 19

Stretching methods for lower back and sacrum pain:

- Rhythmic Breathing (see p. 32)
- Static Stretching (see pp. 32–33)
- PNF Stretching (gently) (see p. 33)

1 hip flexors: knee to chest, stretch 35

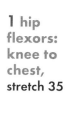
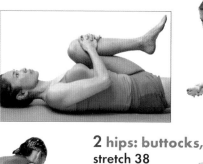

2 hips: buttocks, stretch 38

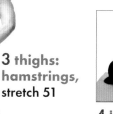

3 thighs: hamstrings, stretch 51

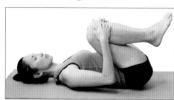

4 lower back: flexion, stretch 11a

Hip

If your pain is in the front of the hip (hip flexors), it may be caused by, for example:

- Simple overuse—repetitive flexing of your hip when you walk, run, or do knee lifts.
- Layering extensive use on top of inadequately stretched hip flexors.

If your pain is on the side of the hip, look into overuse and concentrate on stretch 42. If your pain is in the buttocks area of the hip, it may be caused by, for example:

- Running on a surface that is too hard—such as concrete.
- Prolonged sitting.

Try out this group of hip stretches (plus one for the thighs). As you become familiar with more stretches, you can add to the ones below, or substitute the ones that work best for you.

Stretching methods for hip pain:

- Rhythmic Breathing (see p. 32)
- Static Stretching (see pp. 32–33)
- PNF Stretching (gently) (see p. 33)

Next steps

When the pain condition improves, you can add more intensity to the stretches in this section, or continue your flexibility improvement by adding more intense stretches, for example:

1 thighs: quadriceps, stretch 50

2 hips: buttocks, stretch 40

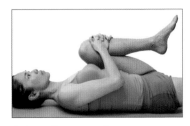

1 hip flexors: knee to chest, stretch 35

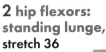

2 hip flexors: standing lunge, stretch 36

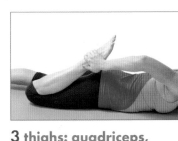

3 thighs: quadriceps, stretch 49

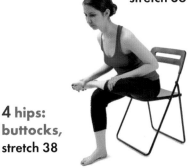

4 hips: buttocks, stretch 38

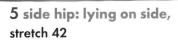

5 side hip: lying on side, stretch 42

Knee

Some possible causes for knee pain could be:

- Muscular imbalance (a) between quadriceps and hamstrings; or (b) among the four quadriceps muscles (see *Thighs*, p. 100, for a fuller explanation).

- Overuse—too much activity without building up to the level of exertion gradually.

- Incorrect form when performing physical activities—such as not lining your knee up over your toes.

- Repetitive movement of the knee or kneeling for long periods.

- Neglecting to warm up before activity.

The following group of stretches will stretch the muscles all around the knee. As with any pain condition (once the pain has subsided enough to enter the stretching phase of recovery), go slowly and gently, feeling your way into each stretch.

Stretching methods for knee pain:

- Rhythmic Breathing (see p. 32)
- Static Stretching (see pp. 32–33)

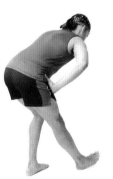

1 thighs: hamstrings, stretch 51

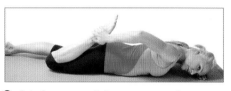

2 thighs: quadriceps, stretch 49

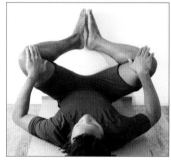

3 inner thighs: feet on wall, stretch 45

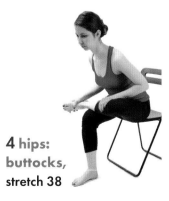

4 hips: buttocks, stretch 38

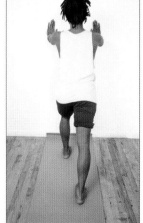

5 calves: floor, leg straight, stretch 54a

Next steps

When the pain condition improves, you can add more intensity to the stretches in this section, or continue your flexibility improvement by adding more intense stretches, for example:

1 thighs: quadriceps, stretch 50

2 hips: buttocks, stretch 40

Stretch to increase range of motion

There is really just one reason to use stretching techniques to increase your range of motion in muscles and joints—it makes doing what you do easier. This applies whether you want to regain a normal ability that has been diminished—perhaps through injury, surgery, or lack of use; whether you want to develop a new ability that you never had; or whether you aspire to the maximum flexibility level of which the human body is capable.

The stretching method you use will change based on your goal (see *Part One: Ways to Stretch*, p. 31). You must adjust the intensity of the felt stretch based on this goal. Naturally, if you are recovering from injury, your initial approach to regaining lost flexibility will be gentler. If your muscles are basically healthy and you are working toward a split, more intensity is called for.

Besides selecting the appropriate method of training to help you reach your stretching goal, there is the question of which stretches will be most helpful. The number of stretches available today is legion—and new ones are being created all the time as people explore more efficient ways to become more flexible. This book is a jumping-off point for you as you start to acquaint yourself with the abundance of stretching tools out there. The guidelines offered in this text can form the groundwork for your stretching education, a solid basis on which you can build further progress.

Part Two: Your Stretch Repertory (see p. 42) provides a basic, necessarily limited repertory of stretches from which to choose as you steadily pursue your desired range-of-motion goals. This is your palette of stretching "colors" from which to select your trusted tools.

This section explores two ideas you can combine when selecting stretches to increase your range of motion:

1 **List of stretches.** For each body area discussed, a stretch sequence lists not only the obvious stretches—that is, stretches under the *Neck* heading to increase neck flexibility—but also stretches for muscular areas you might not associate with getting flexible in the stated area.

2 **Intensity of stretches.** Some stretches are less intense by nature, and don't open your body deeply enough once your flexibility level goes higher. Each pictured sequence starts you off with less intense stretches. If there are more intense stretches you can investigate (within our present stretching universe), they are listed in the *For Added Intensity* box. When you feel ready for a greater stretching challenge, explore those stretches.

Here, we offer suggestions for increasing your range of motion in the Neck, Shoulder, Hamstring/Lower-Back Connection, and Hip Flexors/Quadriceps muscular areas.

Neck

In addition to the five stretches in the Neck section of *Part Two: Your Stretch Repertory* (pp. 45–49), create greater neck range by adding stretches for the front and back of the shoulder. When you are able to relax and open your shoulders, your neck will automatically carry less habitual tension.

The neck is something of a special case. Even if you have no injury or other neck issue, you will want to stay with gentle techniques when working with the neck. It's never good to yank your neck violently around. Always be kind to your cervical vertebrae. Instead of utilizing more intense techniques, provide greater intensity by adding the shoulder stretches.

Stretching methods for increasing range of neck motion:

- Rhythmic Breathing (see p. 32)
- Longer Static Stretching (see pp. 32–33)

For added intensity

1 shoulders: front, stretch 6

2 shoulders: back, stretch 8

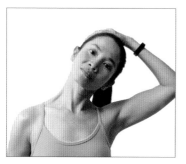

1 neck: side, stretch 1

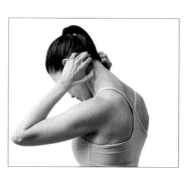

2 neck: back, stretch 2

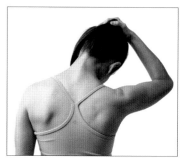

3 neck: back diagonal, stretch 3

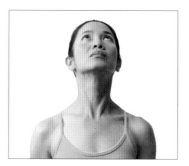

4 neck: front, stretch 4

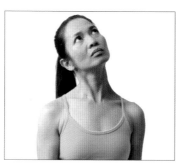

5 neck: front diagonal, stretch 5

Shoulder

The muscle fibers in your chest that are uppermost—closest in location to your shoulders—are addressed in stretch 10b (clavicular = related to the *clavicle*, or collarbone).

Use your own judgment to determine whether stretch 6 or 7 is more intense. Carefully feel your way into each—you will know. This is a matter for individual choice.

Remember not to use stretches 7–9 in the warm-up for swimming. Generally, stretching to gain range of motion is best done either after an intense workout or as an independent workout (after warming up, of course).

Stretching methods for increasing range of shoulder motion:

- Rhythmic Breathing (see p. 32)
- Shorter Static Stretching (see pp. 32–33)
- Longer Static Stretching (see pp. 32–33)

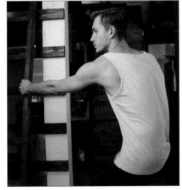

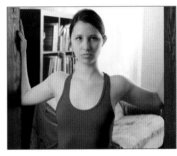

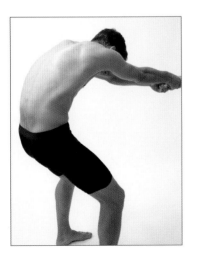

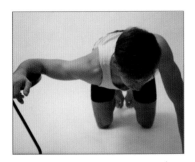

1 shoulders: front, stretch 6

2 shoulders: back, stretch 9

3 chest: below shoulder level, stretch 10b

4 upper back: flexion, stretch 19

For added intensity

1 shoulders: front, stretch 7

2 shoulders: back, stretch 8

Hamstring/lower-back connection

A lovely, functional, open, flexible hamstring/lower-back connection is one of the major casualties of our culture. As a society, we sit—often for long periods of time. Sitting encourages slumping. The lower back and sacrum tuck under; the shoulders round inward; the chin juts out. When muscles don't move, they stiffen. The hamstring and lower-back muscles may get so short that, when we stand up, we cannot lift our knee to 90 degrees. This important muscular connection is definitely an area to address if we want to restore our original range of motion—and go beyond.

The plough is part of the sequence below. It is rightly considered a more intense stretch, and should be practiced with care (see *Part Two:*

Your Stretch Repertory, p. 61). But it is given here as part of a three-stretch progression to open the lower back. Since you will be doing these stretches at a time when you are not moving on to another kind of workout, you can take the time to explore how the felt stretch increases during this lower-back mini-sequence.

Stretching methods for increasing hamstring and lower-back range of motion:

- Rhythmic Breathing (see p. 32)
- Static Stretching (see pp. 32–33)
- PNF Stretching (for hamstring stretches) (see p. 33)

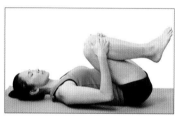

1 lower back: flexion, stretch 11a

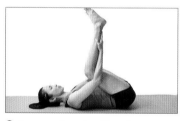

2 lower back: flexion, stretch 11b

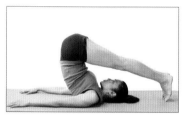

3 lower back: flexion, stretch 11c

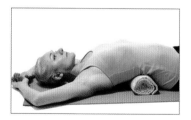

4 lower back: extension, stretch 17

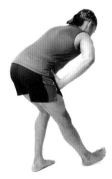

5 thighs: hamstrings, stretch 51

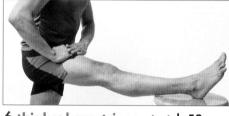

6 thighs: hamstrings, stretch 53

For added intensity

1 lower back: extension, stretch 15

2 thighs: hamstrings, stretch 52

Hip flexors/quadriceps

The hip flexors and quadriceps are related. Stretching the quadriceps is the first step in opening a long muscular line that extends all the way up the front of your body into the deeply seated hip-flexor muscle group. Lengthening this muscular chain counteracts the effects of constant sitting and assists your pelvis to assume its correct lumbar curve.

Stretch 4 below, for the inner thighs, has the legs fully extended (long hip adductors). Although straightening the legs usually makes an inner-thigh stretch more intense, it is possible to get very relaxed while lying on your back with your legs totally supported by the wall—even though they are completely open. You can utilize a long static stretch here—even five minutes. You can even close your eyes and zone out.

When you progress to *For Added Intensity*, it may surprise you that a back-extension stretch can open up the hip flexors and quadriceps area. If you perform this stretch correctly (see *Part Two: Your Stretch Repertory*, p. 67),

your lower back will lengthen in the extended position, and you will also eventually access a stretchy feeling deep into your abdominal area—you're feeling the mysterious psoas muscle.

Stretching methods for increasing hip-flexor and quadriceps range of motion:

- Rhythmic Breathing (see p. 32)
- Longer Static Stretching (see pp. 32–33)
- Gravity—stretch 48 (very heavy legs)
- PNF Stretching—stretches 36, 37, 50, 52 (see p. 33)

For added intensity

1 lower back: extension, stretch 16

2 hip flexors: kneeling lunge, stretch 37

3 thighs: quadriceps, stretch 50

4 inner thighs: kneeling, stretch 46

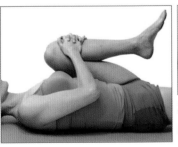

1 hip flexors: knee to chest, stretch 35

2 hip flexors: standing lunge, stretch 36

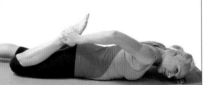

3 thighs: quadriceps, stretch 49

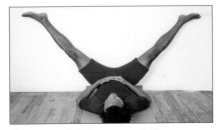

5 inner thighs: straddle, stretch 48

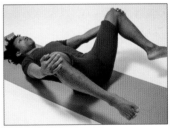

4 inner thighs: knees over hips, stretch 44

The freedom to move easily and gracefully in any direction—without even thinking—is your birthright. If you have lost it you can take it back, with the right tools, concentration, and consistency.

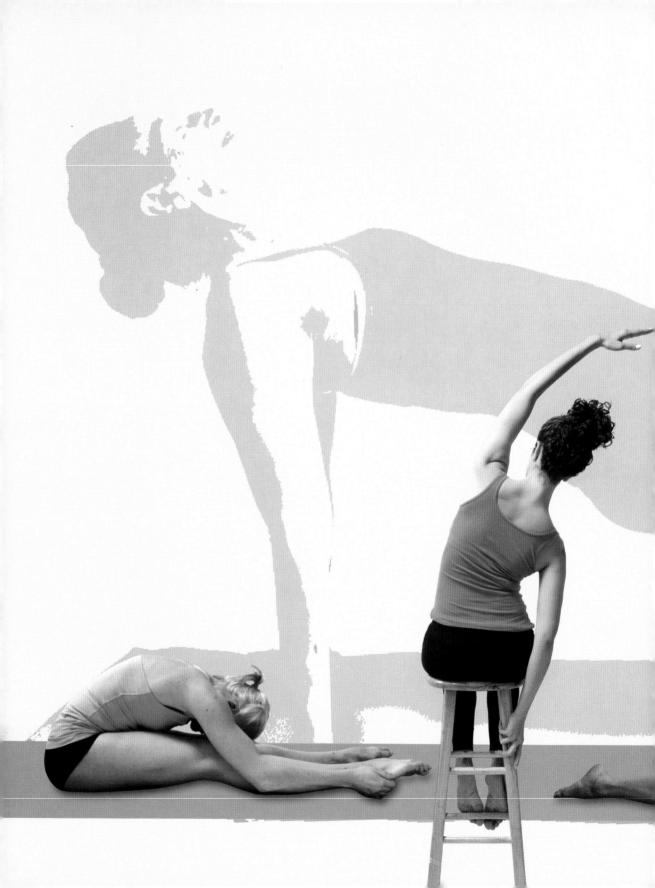

PART FOUR
YOUR FIT AND FLEXIBLE BODY

The stretching experience is necessarily different for each individual. You are a unique person—no one else has precisely your life experience, so no one else has precisely your stretching requirements. This section is the icing on the cake—glimpses of new vistas will open as you create an improved life experience incorporating stretching concepts. Develop what you learned from *Parts Two* and *Three* through considering the ideas in these articles. You no longer have to founder in the dark, wondering what flexibility is all about. Note down ideas that occur to you in odd moments—these flashes of inspiration will form the basis for truly brilliant ways to use stretching as life enhancement.

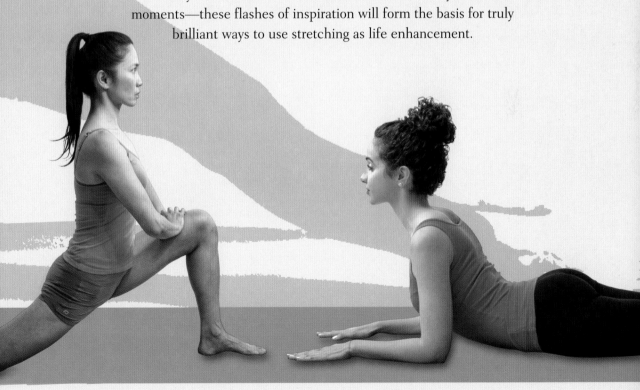

Create your own stretching routines

When I first came to New York City, the greatest city in the world (you can tell I live there), I was a starving artist in graduate school. I frequently found myself dining in your basic generic Chinese restaurant. The menus there were a standing joke among students. They invariably sported two columns of available dishes: Group A and Group B. Several dinner prices were quoted, and for each price you were directed to "choose one from Group A and two from Group B," or various other permutations of that formula.

That idea is a good blueprint for creating your custom stretching routines. You are assembling a flexibility package to match your current intention.

Here are your basic "groups," gathered from topics covered in this book:

Group A: Goals

What is your goal? OR What do you want to accomplish by stretching? OR Why do you want to stretch?

1   Loosen tight muscles. Ask yourself: what muscles feel tight?
    Hint: Tune in to the signals you get from your body. Tight muscles usually occur in the muscles used for the dominant movement patterns of your sport.

2   Relieve an area of pain: what hurts?

3   Relieve stiffness resulting from daily life tasks.

4   Prepare to do a physical activity.

5   Recover after doing a physical activity.

6   Increase range of motion to the level needed for an activity or daily life task.

7   Relax and de-stress.

Group B: Time

How much time do you want to spend stretching?

1   15 minutes

2   30 minutes

3   45 minutes

4   1 hour

5   Unlimited

Group C: Stretches

Which stretches will you include?

1   How many stretches to do: based on the time you have. (Certain breathing-method choices tend to increase time spent in a particular stretch, see *Part One: Using the Tool of Breathing*, p. 34).

2   Which muscles to stretch: based on your goal (see *Part Three: Stretch Sequences*, p. 134).

Group D: Method

Which stretching method will you use?

1   Stretch in Motion

2   Shorter Static Stretching

3   Longer Static Stretching

4   Rhythmic Breathing

5   PNF Stretching

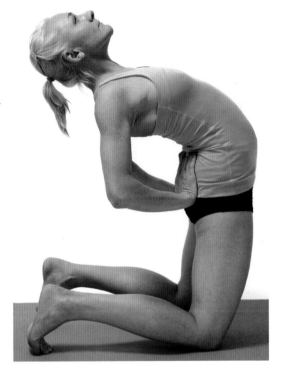

Create your custom routine using the various guidelines discussed in previous sections. What are your priorities for this routine? If the time you have available is the key factor, let that determine the other session parameters. If you can spend more time on stretching, make your goal the starting point.

YOUR STRETCHING "MENU"

GROUP A: GOAL	GROUP B: TIME	GROUP C: STRETCHES	GROUP D: METHOD
Loosen tight muscles	15 minutes	Choose from Part Two based on choices from Groups A and B	Stretch in Motion
Relieve painful area	30 minutes		Shorter Static Stretching
Relieve stiffness	45 minutes		Longer Static Stretching
Prepare for activity	1 hour		Rhythmic Breathing
Recover after activity	Unlimited		PNF Stretching
Increase range of motion			
Relax and de-stress			

Sample flexibility practice plans

This section presents several flexibility training plans, based on the menu model developed in *Create Your Own Stretching Routines*. Below is the menu matrix:

GROUP A: GOAL	GROUP B: TIME	GROUP C: STRETCHES	GROUP D: METHOD
Loosen tight muscles	15 minutes	Choose from Part Two based on Groups A and B	Stretch in Motion
Relieve painful area	30 minutes		Shorter Static Stretching
Relieve stiffness	45 minutes		Longer Static Stretching
Prepare for activity	1 hour		Rhythmic Breathing
Recover after activity	Unlimited		PNF Stretching
Increase range of motion			
Relax and de-stress			

Sample Plan 1: Relieve Painful Area

GROUP A: GOAL	GROUP B: TIME	GROUP C: STRETCHES	GROUP D: METHOD
Relieve knee pain	15 minutes	1. Thighs: hamstrings, stretch 51	Shorter Static Stretching
		2. Thighs: quadriceps, stretch 49	
		3. Inner thighs: feet on wall, stretch 45	
		4. Hips: buttocks, stretch 38	
		54a. Calves: floor, leg straight, stretch 54a	

Comment: you may be able to cycle through these stretches more than once, or spend longer on each.

Creating your plans: Plug in your own specific objectives. Of course, the plans on these pages are simplified, and capable of many permutations, all based on how your body reacts during your session. Here are some possibilities. You may:

- Decide to use several breathing methods.
- Choose two or more goals to address.
- Allocate more time to some stretches.
- Cycle through several stretches more than once.
- Change the order of the stretches.
- Add or remove stretches.

Sample Plan 2: Relieve Stiffness Resulting from Daily Life Tasks

GROUP A: GOAL	GROUP B: TIME	GROUP C: STRETCHES	GROUP D: METHOD
Prolonged sitting	30 minutes	1. Lower-back:flexion, stretch 14	Rhythmic Breathing
		2. Thighs: hamstrings, stretch 53	
		3. Thighs: quadriceps, stretch 49	
		4. Inner thighs, stretch 47	
		5. Hips: buttocks, stretch 38	
		6. Side hip: knee push, stretch 41	
		7. Hip flexors: knee to chest, stretch 35	

Comment: try alternating Rhythmic Breathing with Shorter Static Stretching.

Sample Plan 3: Recover after Doing a Physical Activity

GROUP A: GOAL	GROUP B: TIME	GROUP C: STRETCHES	GROUP D: METHOD
Recover after walking	45 minutes	1. Thighs: hamstrings, stretch 53	Longer Static Stretching
		2. Thighs: quadriceps, stretch 49	
		3. Hip flexors: standing lunge, stretch 36	
		4. Hips: buttocks, stretch 38	
		5. Side hip: knee push, stretch 41	
		6. Calves: leg straight, stretch 55a	
		7. Ankles: extension, stretch 58	
		8. Shoulders: back, stretch 9	

Comment: stretches 38 and 53 lend themselves to PNF Stretching. Also try some Rhythmic Breathing to increase range.

Supporting flexibility: your lifestyle

Lifestyle is a large word that means the way we live. Life is made up of tiny moments, tiny actions that—taken together—weave the fabric of life. Crafting each little moment into an experience that makes us feel a little better adds up. It's the stuff that creates dreams.

When we read a book of fiction, the author often writes from the point of view of "the omniscient observer," the one who stands aside and sees all. If we cultivate that back-of-the-mind point of view as we live our lives, our automatic behaviors will begin to come to light—and with that awareness, the power to change them begins.

Diet

We have heard forever about the concept of *the diet*. In former years, this meant starving to lose weight. Today we know that this does not work. The weight comes off quickly at first but, at the point when the body realizes it is starving, it holds onto body fat to protect itself against famine. This is our human programming, and our fundamental nature wins every time. Our "diet" is a habitual way of eating.

How to change your diet is another Pandora's box—but basically it boils down to two issues:

1   What should you eat?

2   How can you discipline yourself to eat it?

The first question is an individual matter. Some general considerations to assist your deliberations might be:

- Some foods contribute more to health than others: decide which they are. It was said about the famous nutritionist Adelle Davis that she did not put one morsel of food into her mouth that did not support health.
- Are you eating enough to support your activity level? Generally eat more—not less; but eat foods that contribute to better health.

Some profitable dietary research directions might be *The Paleo Diet* and *The Metabolic Typing Diet*—both of which stem from the premise that our bodies have not altered their basic makeup since ancient times. The foods that supported us then still provide optimal nourishment now. Today's soils are nutritionally depleted, so the best organic food is important, as is supplementation, both basic and for specific support.

Often neglected is hydration—plain, life-giving H_2O. Not coffee or tea or vitaminwater®. You have heard the water wisdom of drinking eight glasses a day as a hydration goal. As you become more active, up your water intake. Remember, your body needs constant replenishment of fluids: its composition is 50 per cent to 75 per cent water. Drink all day, as opposed to gulping all at once.

For some insight on question two, see *Get the Stretching Habit*, p. 181. If you figure out how to create one habit, you can create any habit.

Exercise

Reams of information exist on this topic. One premise of this book is: we live in a body that was meant to move. Get it moving. If you hate "exercise," find some movement that you don't classify as exercise and do it. Moving is important for your health. You can see for yourself the ill effects of constant sitting. I know this first hand: sitting for the number of hours it takes to write this book is not a fun experience. My body wants to move. Your lymphatic system has no pump; it depends on muscle movement to push waste products out of your body. Move, move, move!

Weight training is the king of weight-bearing exercise—and hence bone health. If you hate the gym, there are so many ways to incorporate resistive movement into your life. A whole universe of movement is out there—just ripe for you to come along and choose what you want to do.

Sleep

Do but consider what an excellent thing sleep is: it is so inestimable a jewel that, if a tyrant would give his crown for an hour's slumber, it cannot be bought . . .
—*Thomas Dekker, as quoted in* Gaudy Night, *by Dorothy L. Sayers*

Ah, sleep! It is well known that one-third of our lives is spent sleeping. Something the body does so regularly and inevitably is crucial to its health. Sleep is the body's time for system repair and maintenance, and we cannot shortchange it without ill consequences. The cultivation of deep, restful sleep is of paramount importance to a healthy life—and it makes you feel better, too.

Take charge of your own health

As health-care costs rise and medical specializations become ever more separate from the body's composite health, we must step up to the plate, learn to interpret what our bodies are saying, and respond. No one knows your body as well as you do, because no one lives with it as constantly and intimately as you do. We are not used to being our own "doctor," and it may entail quite a learning curve, but in the end—barring drugs for life-threatening situations and surgery to re-attach a limb—there is not much else that we cannot prevent or cure with the right knowledge and some competent alternative practitioners.

Your work

It is a sad present reality that many people make their living doing something they don't enjoy, because we must have money to operate in this society. Spending a number of hours a day in this way has a dampening effect on good health.

The good news is that the world is changing. Opportunities are opening that didn't exist before. Keep your mind open and your ears peeled. People I know have gotten laid off from their corporate jobs—a sign of our times—and have re-invented themselves in novel ways. And they did it building on small daily events.

Plant the seed in your mind that your "work" will do you and others the most good if it feels like playing. Peter Jackson, the director of *The Lord of the Rings* and *The Hobbit*, understands this. His actors "play" for a living. Many times an actor has commented, "And I get paid for doing *this*?"

Just for a moment, lift your nose from the grindstone. Imagining that life can improve prepares the ground for that very thing. It is not stupid to dream your dreams: they can come true.

Fun

The body thrives on routine. That's true. But when routine threatens to become drudgery, we need to inject some balance and spontaneity. It can be a bit scary to skip something you know you should do—especially for your health—but sometimes we need a mini-vacation. When I was studying karate, I remember not wanting to skip a class—even if I was really ill. I was afraid I might never go back because my routine had been disrupted. Have faith: allowing yourself some slack in your pursuit of health does not mean you have no discipline. If you are on your way to the gym, but suddenly a bunch of friends suggests going bowling, maybe that's the moment to loosen the reins a little. Flexibility training starts with your body, but extends into your life.

Remember: what matters to your body and its well-being is your *biological* age, how close you can come to the highest state of health possible. It's a much more uplifting way to think than adopting the all-pervasive emphasis of our culture on chronological age. Try on the concept that "reversing aging" means aligning your body more closely with the buoyant, optimal state of health presented by a 25-year-old human being. It's an adventure with many possible roads to follow on your way there.

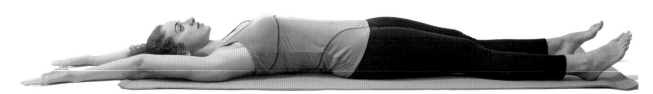

Get the stretching habit

We all have a list umpteen things long that we want to start doing for our health. Change our diet so we eat consistently well; cut out muffins; skip the glass of wine with dinner; get to the gym more; meditate—whatever we are drawn to in the way of healthful practices with the potential to improve how we live.

How many of them do we really adopt, and do them on a regular, continuing basis? We are all too aware that *learning about* how something will benefit us is not the same as *doing* something that will benefit us. So, how do we keep our initial enthusiasm going and create real positive change?

Step 1: awareness

This book is a compendium of suggestions covering many facets of flexibility training. Your reading has probably sparked a number of ideas about how you might like to proceed from here. You might want to look through some sections again to solidify your thoughts, this time making some notes on things you want to incorporate into your own stretching program. Becoming conscious of what your body needs in the way of stretching is one way to make it your own.

Another point worth bearing in mind is that each little moment of your day counts. We all want to get to the big, important things in life, but consistently doing valuable little things will bring us those big ones. Something I tell myself often is, "There is no 'later.'" Life always happens right now.

Step 2: have a plan

If you have an organized plan, you are more likely to implement it. Off-the-cuff, improvised work is fine for an experienced practitioner of stretching who has done it often, has systemized it in his mind, and is familiar with what his body needs and how it reacts. A written plan is no longer necessary. If you are starting out, though, a plan takes away the overwhelming aspect of beginning something, that feeling of "it's too big and I can't face it." Your plan doesn't have to be complicated or lengthy, maybe just some simple strategies that have occurred to you as you read these pages. It could be a few lines you jotted down informally—a guide to pull out when you arrive at the time you've decided on for your first session.

Create Your Own Stretching Routines (see p. 174) presents one way to create an efficient flexibility training plan. That section gives you a blueprint for gathering and arranging the basic ingredients that make up a stretching recipe.

Step 3: get your brain on your side[1]

We are all run by our habits. Our brain creates them to make our lives easier and save brain space. Today we know that the brain is always adapting, based on the shifting input we give it. The brain is a big energy glutton, so it tries to streamline its efforts by making routines into habits. We don't have to think about behaviors the brain has relegated to our autopilot—like walking, what direction our key turns in the lock, turning left on our way to work. That's our brain being efficient. The less we have to think about mundane tasks, the more creative energy we have to come up with brilliant ideas.We can take advantage of this brain behavior and build a stretching habit.

Anatomy of a habit

If we actually examine an action that we classify as a habit, we find this pattern:

CUE → ROUTINE → REWARD

This is called the "habit loop." A real-life example looks like this:

CUE ⟶ ROUTINE ⟶ REWARD

Complete a stressful day → Buy two cookies ⟶ Sweet taste

The real kicker about a habit's power is that it creates a neurological craving. We are not always conscious of this. Habits can form behind our back. But, even without our conscious awareness, when our brain connects cue with reward, it institutes a subconscious craving, and the habit loop engages.

In the case of our real-life example above, we start feeling that our day is not complete without those cookies. Our brain starts looking forward to the reward. We crave it. We may decide that this is not a really great habit and wish to get rid of it. To unravel a habit, first we must identify the craving behind it. We must realize that we want that reward. If we don't bring this knowledge to the surface of our mind, we are in the habit's power.

Create a new habit

We want to make stretch into a habit. Instead of dissipating a non-helpful habit as in the above example, we want to do the reverse and build a new habit. Like this: assemble a cue, a routine, and a reward. Then look for a craving to power the whole thing. Here is an example of a new habit you might construct:

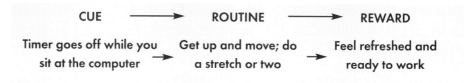

CUE ⟶ ROUTINE ⟶ REWARD

Timer goes off while you sit at the computer → Get up and move; do a stretch or two → Feel refreshed and ready to work

You must go through this cycle as often as it takes to manufacture a craving. The brain must look forward to the good feelings that the reward brings. Then it will start feeling good as soon as the timer goes off. The craving carries you through the routine, time after time.

Lots of people start exercising for reasons important to them. It doesn't matter why you start, but if you want to continue, first set up the habit loop, and then get that craving going. Your cue can be almost anything: a place you're in, the moment of 12:00 noon, an action you do. Same with the reward: it will be something uniquely personal to you. Maybe you watch your favorite TV show; maybe you eat some delicious organic raspberries; maybe you treat yourself to a long, hot soak. Maybe you just feel satisfied with yourself because you did something you know will improve your life.

There's your habit loop. Then the trick is to get your brain to start looking for the good feeling triggered by your chosen reward—make the craving happen. When the behavior feels automatic, you know you've got it. When you feel something is missing because you skipped that behavior, you know you will return to it even if you miss a day. I began practicing the piano when I was seven years old. I did it for so many years that, even today, when I don't practice, I always feel that something is missing from my day. That's a habit.

Revise an existing habit

Another way to get good habits going is to keep the same cue and reward, but revise the routine in the middle. Studies show that you can never really eliminate a habit. Duhigg calls this the "Golden Rule of habit change." So, build on habits you already have. My friends Vinny and Sheila did that quite successfully.

Habit change case 1: Vinny's Hip Flexors. Vinny is a spin instructor with an office job. He ends up with very tight hip flexors, but is short on time. When he was living in a very small apartment, he had a chair sitting right outside his bathroom door. Every time he brushed his teeth at night, he pushed the chair into the bathroom, lifted his foot behind him onto the chair as he stood at the sink, and did a hip-flexor stretch—one minute on a side—while he brushed his teeth for two minutes. He added a new behavior onto an already existing habit loop.

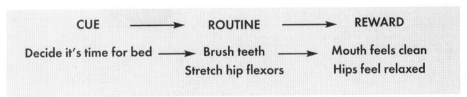

CUE	→	ROUTINE	→	REWARD
Decide it's time for bed	→	Brush teeth	→	Mouth feels clean
		Stretch hip flexors		Hips feel relaxed

Habit change case 2: Sheila's Pliés. Sheila is a singer and dancer. When she was healing a broken ankle, she needed to strengthen the muscles in her foot and ankle before returning to dance class. Every time she did the dishes, she worked the muscles of her legs and feet through plié/relevé. All the while she washed her dishes (mindless activity). She inserted a new behavior into a habit loop she already had.

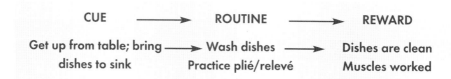

Study your habits. Find out how you can create one or adapt one. You'll soon be stretching on a regular basis.

Further study: flexibility resources

The pursuit of flexibility is a worthy—even necessary—life goal, whether you want to get out of pain, play your favorite sport with ease forever, get yourself a split, or just keep your body healthy and moving throughout your whole life. Stretching is one way to help get you there, and that is the approach I have taken in this book. Some other ideas that blend well for flexibility were presented earlier in this section (see *Supporting Flexibility: Your Lifestyle*, p. 178). Many other health modalities exist. Together with the practice of stretching, a judicious selection of these can produce a synergistic effect on your flexibility progress.

Here I've listed some of my favorites. A full list would be as long as your flexible body, but I have personally experienced the disciplines below, to one degree or another—either through studying the modality and becoming a certified professional myself, or by working with skilled specialists in these areas. Consult the *Bibliography* (see p. 187) for more places to look as you embark on your quest for the flexible life.

- **Massage.** The benefits of massage are well known; a partial list includes trigger-point release, easing muscular tension and spasm, and deep relaxation. Massage can be pricey, so many people who should do it regularly (like me!) don't. To help offset this, consider learning a method of self-massage to prolong the effects of your professional session—very effective as well. Practicing the MELT Method® technique (described opposite) also helps tide you over to your next massage or other bodywork session. Sheila Wormer is an outstanding massage therapist with a practice in New York City. She is qualified in the following modalities: deep tissue, Thai, and lymphatic drainage massage; assisted stretching; reflexology; The Radiance Technique; and Reiki. Contact her by e-mail at: sheila.wormer@gmail.com.

- **The MELT Method®.** "Active, pain-free living for a lifetime" is the MELT slogan. Developed by Sue Hitzmann, MELT employs self-treatment techniques that calm the stress response of your nervous system and hydrate your connective tissue. It is soundly based on current scientific research. Once you learn the techniques from a qualified instructor, you have some effective tools for getting yourself out of pain, increasing your flexibility level, and just generally feeling better. MELT makes use of unique small balls to treat hands and feet, and a specialized soft roller for the rest of the body. I am a certified practitioner of The MELT Method®, and the equipment and bestselling book are available through my website: www.lindasarts.com. For more in-depth information about MELT, visit www.meltmethod.com.

- **Gyrokinesis®.** This is a method of movement/exercise developed by former dancer Juliu Horvath (www.gyrotonic.com). It is a wonderful way to teach your back to rediscover its full movement capabilities—which many bodies today have forgotten. It uses circular and flowing movements; the back acquires ease and fluidity of motion as it loses stiffness. The use of the breath is pivotal to the technique. It's great for relieving back pain, and works well for those with herniated discs and scoliosis. I am a certified instructor of Gyrokinesis®.

- **Aromatherapy.** This is indeed a delightful way to assist your body to open up. A therapist can custom-blend a massage oil for you, precisely matched to your personal emotional and mental makeup. It will contain precious essences extracted from fragrant plant material of various species—from flowers, leaves, bark, wood, roots, fruit peel, or sometimes the entire plant. Complementing stretching with a local self-massage (see *Massage,* opposite) will add a fuller dimension to your stretching practice. Inhalation of marvelous scents can lend flexibility to your mind—which then translates to your body. I hold an aromatherapy certificate from the Australasian College of Health Sciences. My long-time, very knowledgeable supplier of pure organic or wildcrafted essential oils is Mynou De Mey. She has a network of distributors worldwide and can obtain the finest oils offered in the field. Contact her by e-mail at: mynou101@gmail.com.

- **Acupuncture.** This is a well-known way to relieve pain, which utilizes the Chinese medicine system of diagnosis and treatment. It can be an effective adjunct to a well-rounded stretching program. Finding the right "fit" between you and your specialist can be tricky. To supplement your acupuncture sessions, ask your professional for a few points you can massage using the related *acupressure* technique, which allows you to promote your own healing. An excellent New York City-based acupuncturist is Evelyn Li. Contact her by e-mail at ejli.lac@gmail.com.

- **The Alexander Technique.** This is the posture-improving technique par excellence. I have studied with several practitioners over a number of years. One's body can absolutely assimilate this method and make it an intrinsic part of its natural way of moving. A superb Alexander teacher in New York City is Brooke Lieb, Senior Faculty and Director of Teacher Training at the American Center for the Alexander Technique (ACAT). Contact her at: www.brookelieb.com. For more information on the Alexander Technique, visit www.acatnyc.org.

List of muscles

In *Part Two: Your Stretch Repertory*, the muscles illustrated are those that could be easily drawn on the photographic views of the stretches. For a list of additional muscles stretching in each position but not shown, see below (by stretch number):

1. Anterior scalene, splenius capitis.
2. Longissimus capitis, obliquus semispinalis capitis, capitis inferior, rectus capitis posterior major, longissimus cervicis, semispinalis cervicis, interspinales cervicis.
3. Splenius capitis, longissimus capitis, splenius cervicis, longissimus cervicis, semispinalis cervicis, levator scapulae, posterior and medial scalenes, rectus capitis posterior major, obliquus capitis inferior.
4. Longus colli (inferior and superior oblique), anterior scalene.
5. Longus colli (inferior and superior oblique), anterior scalene.
6. Pectoralis minor.
7. Pectoralis minor.
8. Rhomboids.
11c. Spinalis, multifidi, semimembranosus.
15. Spinalis cervicis, spinalis thoracis, semispinalis capitis, semispinalis cervicis, semispinalis thoracis, rotatores breves and longi, interspinales cervicis, interspinales lumborum, intertransversarii laterales lumborum, intertransversarii mediales lumborum, iliopsoas (iliacus, psoas major and minor), external and internal obliques.
16. Spinalis cervicis, semispinalis cervicis, semispinalis thoracis, multifidi, rotatores breves and longi, interspinales cervicis, interspinales lumborum, intertransversarii laterales lumborum, intertransversarii mediales lumborum, iliopsoas (iliacus, psoas major and minor), tensor fascia lata, rectus femoris, sartorius, .external and internal obliques, rectus abdominis.
17. Semispinalis thoracis, multifidi, rotatores breves and longi, interspinales lumborum, intertransversarii laterales lumborum, intertransversarii mediales lumborum, internal oblique.
20. Spinalis thoracis, semispinalis capitis (medial fascicle), semispinalis cervicis, semispinalis thoracis, rotatores breves and longi, intertransversarii mediales lumborum, internal oblique.
21. Spinalis thoracis, semispinalis capitis (medial fascicle), semispinalis cervicis, semispinalis thoracis, rotatores breves and longi, intertransversarii mediales lumborum, internal oblique.
22. Spinalis cervicis, spinalis thoracis, semispinalis capitis, semispinalis cervicis, semispinalis thoracis, rotatores breves and longi, interspinales cervicis, interspinales lumborum, intertransversarii laterales lumborum, intertransversarii mediales lumborum, internal oblique.
23. Spinalis thoracis, semispinalis thoracis, rotatores breves and longi, interspinales, intertransversarii, internal oblique, transversus abdominis, quadratus lumborum.
24a, b. Spinalis thoracis, semispinalis thoracis, multifidi, rotatores breves and longi, interspinales, intertransversarii, gluteus minimus (knee lower), internal oblique, transversus abdominis.
24c. Iliocostalis, longissimus thoracis, spinalis thoracis, semispinalis thoracis, multifidi, rotatores breves and longi,

interspinales, intertransversarii, external and internal obliques, transversus abdominis.
25. Internal oblique.
26. Internal oblique.
27. Anconeus.
28. Anconeus.
31. Flexor carpi ulnaris, palmarus longus, flexor carpi radialis.
32. Extensor digiti minimi, extensor carpi radialis brevis, extensor carpi radialis longus, abductor pollicis longus.
33. Flexor digitorum superficialis, flexor digitorum profundus, opponens pollicis, abductor pollicis brevis, flexor pollicis brevis, opponens digiti minimi, abductor digiti minimi.
34. Extensor indicis, dorsal interossei.
35. Tensor fascia lata, sartorius.
Note: The piriformis, one of the deep six external hip rotators, is an important muscle that stretches in each of stretches 38 through 40. Because of its position deep within the body, the illustrator was not able to draw it on the photographic views shown.
38. Obturator externus, quadratus femoris, piriformis.
39. Piriformis, gemellus superior and inferior, obturator externus and internus, quadratus femoris.
40. Piriformis.
41. Quadratus lumborum.
43. Gluteus minimus.
49. Vastus intermedius, vastus medialis.
50. Vastus intermedius, vastus medialis.
53. Semimembranosus, semitendinosus.
54a, b. Plantaris, popliteus, peroneus longus and brevis, tibialis posterior.
54c. Plantaris, popliteus, peroneus longus and brevis.
55a. Gastrocnemius, Achilles tendon, plantaris. popliteus, peroneus longus and brevis.
55b. Peroneus longus and brevis, tibialis posterior, flexor digitorum longus.
56. Abductor hallucis, lumbricals, flexor digiti minimi brevis, adductor hallucis, flexor hallucis brevis, plantar interossei, dorsal interossei.
57. Extensor hallucis brevis.
58. Peroneus tertius, extensor digitorum brevis, extensor hallucis brevis, extensor hallucis longus, tibialis anterior.
60. Multifidi, semimembranosus, semitendinosus.
61. Multifidi.
62. Iliocostalis lumborum, longissimus, spinalis, multifidi, biceps femoris (short and long heads), pectineus.
63. Biceps femoris (short and long heads), iliopsoas (iliacus, psoas major and minor), sartorius, iliocostalis lumborum, multifidi, interspinales lumborum, intertransversarii laterales lumborum, intertransversarii mediales lumborum.
64. Longissimus cervicis, spinalis cervicis, semispinalis capitis, semispinalis cervicis, semispinalis thoracis, multifidi, rotatores breves and longi, interspinales cervicis, interspinales lumborum, intertransversarii laterales lumborum, intertransversarii mediales lumborum, pectoralis minor, iliopsoas (iliacus, psoas major and minor), sartorius, internal oblique.

Notes

Introduction
1. Brad Walker, *The Anatomy of Stretching: Your Illustrated Guide to Flexibility and Injury Rehabilitation*, 2nd ed.

Part One
1. Michael J. Alter, *Science of Stretching* (Champaign, IL: Human Kinetics,1988), 6.
2. Ann and Chris Frederick, *Stretch to Win: Flexibility for Improved Speed, Power, and Agility* (Champaign, IL: Human Kinetics, 2006), 181.
3. Maxwell Maltz, *Psycho-Cybernetics: A New Way to Get More Living Out of Life* (New York: Simon & Schuster, 1960), ix. Numerous later editions are available. The principles set forth in this book have been widely adapted for use in athletic training.
4. Frederick and Frederick, *Stretch to Win*, 180–81.

Part Three
1. Video illustrating how to execute dynamic shoulder warm-ups: www.usaswimming.org/. Search for "dynamic shoulder warm-up."
2. PDF file containing expanded information about swimming shoulder-stretching protocols: www.usmsswimmer.com/201001/swimmer_stretching.pdf.

Part Four
1. The material in this section is adapted from Charles Duhigg, *The Power of Habit: Why We Do What We Do in Life and Business* (New York: Random House, 2012).

Bibliography

Under "Books and Journal Articles" you will find all the books and articles either specifically referred to in footnotes or consulted while writing this work. Should you wish to pursue an area in depth, I have also included a number of sources that expand on the concepts developed in the text. The entries under "Web Sites" generally make apparent what information can be found at the listed URL. If there is no article title for the entry, there is a brief identifier at the end of the citation. "Other Sources" are those outside the other categories.

Books and Journal Articles
Alter, Michael J. *Science of Stretching*. Champaign, IL: Human Kinetics, 1988.

Anderson, Bob. *Stretching*. 30th anniversary ed. Bolinas, CA: Shelter Publications, Inc., 2010.

Batmanghelidj, F. *Your Body's Many Cries for Water: You're Not Sick; You're Thirsty; Don't Treat Thirst with Medications*, 3rd ed. Vienna: Global Health Solutions, 2008.

Battaglia, Salvatore. *The Complete Guide to Aromatherapy*, 2nd ed. Brisbane, Australia: The International Centre of Holistic Aromatherapy, 2003.

Clark, Linda, and Yvonne Martine. *Health, Youth, and Beauty through Color Breathing*. Berkeley: Celestial Arts Publishing Co., 1995.

Cordain, Loren. *The Paleo Diet: Lose Weight and Get Healthy by Eating the Foods You Were Designed to Eat*. Hoboken, NJ: John Wiley & Sons, Ltd., 2010.

Davis, Adelle. *Let's Eat Right to Keep Fit*, rev. ed. New York: Signet Books, 1970.

Delavier, Frédéric, Jean-Pierre Clémenceau, and Michael Gundill. *Delavier's Stretching Anatomy*. Champaign, IL: Human Kinetics, 2010.

Dement, William C., and Christopher Vaughn. *The Promise of Sleep: A Pioneer in Sleep Medicine Explores the Vital Connection between Health, Happiness, and a Good Night's Sleep*. New York: Random House, Inc., 2000.

Duhigg, Charles. *The Power of Habit: Why We Do What We Do in Life and Business*. New York: Random House Trade Paperbacks, 2014. First published 2012 by Random House.

Frederick, Ann, and Chris Frederick. *Stretch to Win: Flexibility for Improved Speed, Power, and Agility*. Champaign, IL: Human Kinetics, 2006.

Gray, Henry. *Anatomy, Descriptive and Surgical*. Edited by T. Pickering Pick and Robert Howden. Philadelphia: Courage Books, 1974. First published 1901 by Lea Brothers, Philadelphia. Gray's *Anatomy* publication history: http://en.wikipedia.org/wiki/Gray%27s_Anatomy. Title page of original 1901 edition: https://archive.org/details/anatomydescripti1901gray.

Hitzmann, Sue. *The MELT Method: A Breakthrough Self-Treatment System to Eliminate Chronic Pain, Erase the Signs of Aging, and Feel Fantastic in Just 10 Minutes a Day!* New York: HarperOne, 2013.

Hoppenfeld, Stanley. *Physical Examination of the Spine and Extremities*. Norwalk, CT: Appleton-Century-Crofts, 1976.

Kapit, Wynn, and Lawrence M. Elson. *The Anatomy Coloring Book*. 2nd ed. New York: HarperCollins College Publishers, 1993.

Lally, Phillippa, Cornelia H. M. van Jaarsveld, Henry W. W. Potts, and Jane Wardle. "How Are Habits Formed: Modelling Habit Formation in the Real World." *European Journal of Social Psychology* 40, no. 6 (2010): 998–1009. doi:10.1002/ejsp.674.

Nelson, Arnold G., and Jouko Kokkonen. *Stretching Anatomy: Your Illustrated Guide to Improving Flexibility and Muscular Strength*. Champaign, IL: Human Kinetics, 2007.

Osar, Evan. *Corrective Exercise Solutions to Common Hip and Shoulder Dysfunction*. Aptos, CA: On Target Publications, 2012.

Ramsay, Craig. *Anatomy of Stretching: A Guide to Increasing Your Flexibility*. San Diego: Thunder Bay Press, 2012.

Sasaki, Kotaro, and Richard R. Neptune. "Differences in Muscle Function during Walking and Running at the Same Speed." *Journal of Biomechanics* 39 (2006). doi:10.1016/j.jbiomech.2005.06.019.

Sayers, Dorothy L. *Gaudy Night*. London: The Folio Society, 1998. First published 1935 by Victor Gollancz, Ltd.

Tourles, Stephanie. *Natural Foot Care: Herbal Treatments, Massage, and Exercises for Healthy Feet*. Pownal, Vermont: Storey Books, 1998.

Walker, Brad. *The Anatomy of Stretching: Your Illustrated Guide to Flexibility and Injury Rehabilitation*, 2nd ed. Berkeley: North Atlantic Books, 2011.

Weinberg, Norma Pasekoff. *Natural Hand Care: Herbal Treatments and Simple Techniques for Healthy Hands and Nails*. Pownal, Vermont: Storey Books, 1998.

Wolcott, William L., and Trish Fahey. *The Metabolic Typing Diet*. New York: Doubleday, 2000.

Worwood, Valerie Ann. *The Complete Book of Essential Oils and Aromatherapy*. San Rafael, CA: New World Library, 1991.

Websites

The Ballet Bag. "Bag of Steps: Eight Positions/." May 20, 2009. www.theballetbag.com/2009/05/20/bag-of-steps-eight-positions.
How to align your hips at the barre.

"Color Breathing Exercise for Stress Relief." Milwaukee Portal. Accessed February 20, 2015. http://city.milwaukee.gov/ImageLibrary/User/jkamme/EAP/Info-Library/MentalHealth_5QuickStressReduc.pdf.

Do-It-Yourself Joint Pain Relief. Gary Crowley. Accessed February 20, 2015. www.do-it-yourself-joint-pain-relief.com/subscapularis-stretch.html.
Subscapularis *stretch*.

"How Leg Workouts for Runners Work." John Kelly. July 14, 2010. http://adventure.howstuffworks.com/outdoor-activities/running/training/leg-workouts-for-runners1.htm.
Muscles used in running.

"How Long Can a Person Survive without Water?" Corey Binns. November 30, 2012. www.livescience.com/32320-how-long-can-a-person-survive-without-water.html.

"How Long Can the Brain Be without Oxygen before Brain Damage?" Erin J. Hill. Last modified February 9, 2015. www.wisegeek.org/how-long-can-the-brain-be-without-oxygen-before-brain-damage.htm.

"How Long Can You Hold Your Breath? The Physical Effects of Training for World Records and Free Diving." Brian Palmer. Last updated November 19, 2013. www.slate.com/articles/health_and_science/explainer/2013/11/nicholas_mevoli_freediving_death_what_happens_to_people_who_practice_holding.html.

"How Much of Your Body Is Water?" Anne Marie Helmenstine. October 18, 2014. http://chemistry.about.com/od/waterchemistry/f/How-Much-Of-Your-Body-Is-Water.htm.

"Multifidus Muscle." Sam Visnic. Instructional video. Accessed February 20, 2015. www.youtube.com/watch?v=XBDz6YUz7xk.

"Navel." Wikipedia. Last modified February 16, 2015. http://en.wikipedia.org/wiki/Navel.
Vertebrae opposite the navel.

"Neurons That Fire Together Wire Together." Curt Thompson, July 14, 2010. www.beingknown.com/2010/07/neurons-that-fire-together-wire-together.

"Rotator Cuff Series: *Supraspinatus*/Middle Deltoid." Kit Laughlin. November 22, 2011. www.youtube.com/watch?v=1Pl_p64l_ps.
How to stretch the supraspinatus *muscle.*

"Save Yourself from IT Band Syndrome!" Paul Ingraham. Introduction to e-book, last updated September 23, 2014. www.painscience.com/tutorials/iliotibial-band-syndrome.php.

"Stretching: Expert Advice on the Art of Loosening Up." Keith Scott. Accessed February 20, 2015. http://www.mensfitness.com/training/build-muscle/stretching.
Scientific studies exhibit varied opinions about stretching effects.

"Stretching: the Truth." Thomas Michaud. Accessed February 20, 2015. www.takethemagicstep.com/coaching/families/health-management/stretching-the-truth.
Cites research on whether or not stretching weakens muscles.

"The Truth about Stretching." Sonya Collins. February 25, 2014. www.webmd.com/fitness-exercise/guide/how-to-stretch?page=1.
When to stretch.

"The Vertebral Column: Anatomy/Positioning." Quizlet. Accessed February 20, 2015. http://quizlet.com/9980565/the-vertebral-column-anatomypositioning-flash-cards/.
Vertebrae opposite the navel.

"What Muscles Does Biking Use?" Peggy Hansen. Accessed February 20, 2015. www.trails.com/list_931_what-muscles-does-biking-use.html.

"Which Muscles Does Biking Work?" Jasmine Myers. Accessed February 20, 2015. http://exercise.lovetoknow.com/What_Muscles_Does_Biking_Work.

Other Sources

Chek, Paul. "Flatten Your Abs Forever." Lecture DVD, two hours. Accessed February 20, 2015. https://chekandpps.infusionsoft.com/app/storeFront/showProductDetail?productId=152.

Marinell, LeRoy, Waddy Wachtel, and Warren Zevon. "Werewolves of London." From the album *Excitable Boy*. Asylum Records, 1978. Performed by Warren Zevon.

Welland, Colin (screenplay). *Chariots of Fire*. Film. David Puttnam (producer), 1981.

Index

Acknowledgments

When I read an author's "Acknowledgments" section, I always see something like "many people were involved in this project and no one writes a book alone." This has always annoyed me—who wrote the book anyway? However, now that I have some inkling of what is involved in bringing such a monumental undertaking to fruition, I'm afraid I'm going to say exactly the same thing.

I feel as though this is my Academy Award night and I'm giving my acceptance speech. Those silly recipients always have to be pulled off the stage with a hook because they just can't stop thanking people—often with tears in their eyes. But I have to admit now that I feel just like them. Even without searching in my memory—and though I'm probably missing a bunch of people I should be mentioning—there are scores of folks I must thank for what they did to help me on this project. Here goes.

With gratitude to:
Kristine Pidkameny, for championing my cause with CICO Books because she believed so strongly in my ability to share my knowledge about flexibility with others. I owe to her this astonishing opportunity to publish a book. She also came up with the title.

Cindy Richards, the Publisher at CICO Books, for her vote of confidence to a new author; Dawn Bates, Managing Editor, Sally Powell, Art Director, and the rest of the staff at CICO Books, for their concerted efforts to make this project a success.

The wonderful fitness professionals with whom I have studied, for helping me mold my athletic abilities over many years: Dale Stine—aerobic dance; Tom deFlora, James Windus, Rafael Ulloa, and Kevin Richardson—bodybuilding; Nina Ries—yoga therapy; Kirill Matveev, Natalya Stavro, and Setsuko Maruhashi—ballet; Young-Ah Kim, Billy Macagnone, and Leslie Davenport—Gyrokinesis; and Ekaterina Sknarina—rhythmic gymnastics.

Marc Rudin, D.C., my chiropractor, for his willingness to allow me to bounce ideas off him, for his encouragement of my sometimes-oddball stretching point of view, and for his constant, uplifting appreciation for what I'm trying to achieve in my life.

The medical and fitness professionals of my wider network, some of whom I have only met virtually, for their generosity with time and information. They contributed their expertise to answer my questions about "which muscles stretch when": Gary Crowley; Paul Ingraham; Rick Kaselj; Kit Laughlin; Jenice Mattek; Evan Osar, D.C.; and Sam Visnic.

My friends and fitness colleagues who contributed information on subjects of which I am less than mistress: Vinny Bonanno, for the yoga style list and the toothbrushing story; Sheryl Dluginski, for the Lizard Pose; Michael Mcardle, for yoga warm-up ideas; Greg Peck, for sport-stretching information; Liane Plane, for a lovely breathing suggestion; Merek Royce Press, my long-suffering web technician, for

intelligent tennis information from a non-professional player's point of view, and for rescuing me from a computer virus during my last frantic week of writing; and James Windus, LMHC, my weight trainer from lifetimes ago, for helping me clarify the research approach I was taking.

Evelyn Li, L.Ac., L.M.T., my friend and gifted acupuncturist, for alerting me to the enormity of the question: "which muscles are stretching when?"

My friends and fitness colleagues, for contributing their time and talents as photographic models: Victor Cabezas; Solange Gomez; Lean Lim; and Ekaterina Sknarina.

My group fitness supervisors, for ongoing opportunities to develop as a teacher: Maryann Donner, Group Fitness Director, New York Health & Racquet Clubs; and Lennie McKenzie, Group Fitness Supervisor, Equitable Athletic & Swim Club.

Helpers in the wings: Mynou De Mey, for the inside scoop on the aromatherapy community; Virginia Doran, for her face massage technique; Sue Hitzmann, author of the best-selling *The MELT Method*, for clueing me in about getting published; Krista Kavilo, for streamlining the text review; and Ahbi Nishman, for the great makeup.

My rooting section: Gregg Hubbard, for brainstorming PR ideas with me; Amy McGlinn, for pure, foot-stomping cheerleading; Suzanne Ruffa, for saying umpteen times, "It's so exciting!"; Nuri Wernick, for her enthusiastic promotional savvy. Her voice reverberates in my ear, sending me to "YouTube, YouTube"!; Sheila Wormer, for her unfailing cheerfulness, readiness to listen, and delightful plié story; and my 56th Street fitness family at NYHRC, for always being there and making me feel that I am one of you.

Rob Zeller, photographer and artist, for his beautiful photographs and illustrations. Text and art take up comparable space in a work like this, and must harmonize and flow together well. Rob made sure they did.

The additional photographic models, for their patience and good humor: Jamal Clarke, Melissa Perry, and Dmitry Prokofyev.

All the students who have attended my fitness classes over the last 22 years, for the opportunity to touch your lives, and for allowing me to hone my teaching practice by working with you.

My marvelous sister Jane Hauptman, for being the familiar, comforting spirit of my growing-up days, when we shared the attic bedroom at 522 6th Avenue; for speaking my literary language with me; and for tirelessly bestowing upon me her voice of reason and calm reassurance when I was freaking out at midnight: "Don't panic. You can do it." I love you, Janie. Take star billing.